The Beer Diet (A L

To Jim & the crew
The Hungry Monk —
Still the **BEST** craft
beer bar in the East Valley!
Thanx for years of friendship.

Vo Izzo

The Beer Diet

(A Brew Story)

Written by Evo Terra
and
Dr. Terry Simpson

Copyedited by Karen Conlin

ISBN: 978-1493666935

Contents

Introduction

By Charlie "the Beer Guy" Cavanaugh Toft
October 2013

Three hundred years ago, monastic brewers in Munich refused to give up beer during Lent. Indeed, they promoted beer to their sole source of sustenance during their month-long fasts, inventing a calorie-rich style called the dopplebock to stave off starvation while getting their brew on at the same time.

As a lifelong lover of the art, science, history, and culture of beer and brewing, I have always looked on these monks with admiration and more than a little envy. Imagine a month of literally nothing but beer drinking, officially sanctioned–even applauded–by society!

But sadly, I'm not a Bavarian monk. I've got a job teaching highschool science. I've got a wife and two kids. I've got, you know, responsibilities.

Not so much my friend Evo Terra. What Evo has–in glorious, overflowing quantities–is lust for life.

Evo and I met eight years ago by way of podcasting. Specifically, he was producing several podcasts and I was listening to them. I was drawn to this hilariously snarky loudmouth, who was nonetheless clearly intelligent and at times even insightful, as he turned his unique blend of sarcasm and enthusiasm to topics of all kinds. Much of the discussion on his shows surrounded movies, TV, books, and other media–mostly science fiction and fantasy–but imagine my delight and surprise when one day I heard him crack a beer on the air (or rather, on the pod).

I believe it was a Guinness, the Irish equivalent of Budweiser. He proceeded to wax rhapsodic about it, at which point I started to cringe behind my earbuds. Here was a bright and charismatic potential spokesperson for quality beer praising mass-produced swill. Seeing that the podcast was produced locally, I immediately jumped on the email and requested permission to drop by with some craft beer and set things right. I now know Evo is an inveterate neophile, but all those years ago I was stunned that he acquiesced, inviting a stranger into the studio and giving him microphone time to talk beer.

I eventually became a regular, acquiring the nom de plume "Charlie the Beer Guy" and soon had a podcast of my own called "Speaking of Beer," produced with Evo's generous support. And thus I fell into his carefully laid trap. You see, I thought I was expressing my passion for beer and indulging my compulsive drive to educate and enlighten. In fact, what I was doing was systematically transferring all of my beer knowledge into the mind of Evo Terra.

And over the years the student has grown to eclipse the master. As it turns out, in that crazy unpredictable way the Universe goes, life has forced me to give up my beer-centered lifestyle altogether. So, now Evo carries my torch of cervesophilia, his focus ever on quality and craftsmanship, as it should be.

Which brings us to the experiment detailed in the pages to follow. Like myself, Evo clearly envied those monks from centuries ago. Unlike myself, however, he took on the challenge of a month of beer with tremendous joie de vivre. And he added sausage.

And–somehow–made the whole thing about science.

At the time I was impressed enough with Evo's project to have a go at it myself. Given that I cross paths with Evo in this book, I won't spoil things with details on how that turned out, but regardless, it was a blast following his progress in real time, as it was reliving those memories reading this time capsule from that month.

One story that jumped out at me was his recounting of a Beer Diet lunch we shared in the early going. I didn't notice it at the time, but it turns out one of the beers we were served was a rich Bavarian lager called Celebrator. Fittingly, that's the selfsame doppelbock that nourished those Munich brothers way back when.

In addition to being a fascinating and entertaining dietary experiment, the Beer Diet turns out to be a terrific path to vicarious wish fulfillment. Thanks to my friend Evo, I got my monastic moment after all.

Prost!

I

Prep Work

"Plan, plan… I need a plan." – Hedley
Lamarr

1

The Beer Diet: The Beginning

Sept 26, 2011

Did you hear the one about the guy whose diet consisted of nothing but craft beer and sausage for the month of October?

Me either. But you're about to. Me too, since I'm *the guy*. That's right. During the month of October 2011, my calories will only come from craft beer and sausage. Yeah. I'm serious. And yes, I'm being monitored by a physician.

You see, I like craft beer. A lot. I've been pondering the idea of a "beer fast" for sometime now and am ready to give it a shot. The month that Oktoberfest takes its name from seems a good time to try it. And unlike those who've attempted to re-create the monks' habit of fasting with beer only, I'm playing fully into the spirit of the season, adding sausage to my diet. Hey, my doctor says I need a little protein to retain muscle mass, and who the hell am I to argue with a doctor? Especially when he says I need to eat sausage!

The Plan

My plan is pretty simple and is as follows:

- **Keep the protein intake to about 30 grams daily.**
  That's not a lot. According to MyFitnessPal, that's about
  one big sausage link.
- **Drink beer.** I only drink quality craft beers, and they
  bring their own protein to the party. Not much, but
  some.
- **Keep total calories around 1700 per day.** With the
  kind of beer I drink, that roughly becomes 5 or 6 beers,
  plus a sausage. A day. Every day. Morning. Noon. Night.
  Oh, and three other times. Life is good.

Then it's rinse and repeat for the entire month of October. Which,
with client meetings and business-related travel, will be interesting. But I'm nothing if not tenacious.Yes, I'll drink plenty of water.
And I'm rather addicted to my morning *yerba mate,* so that's continuing. But other foods are out. Call me crazy.

Follow my progress

I'm also reaching out to the fine folks that run Untappd, a beer
check-in app that I've been evangelizing for a while. I'm hoping to
convince them to make a special badge for people who drink along
with me. No, I don't expect you to try to keep up. But maybe you'll
win a badge if you drink one beer with me each day, or maybe 5
of the beers I check into each week. Not quite sure how that all
works. I'll leave it to them.

Untappd is the best place to keep up with my daily drinking,
though I will try to post a daily re-cap on my blog as well. I''ve
already secured the http://brewdiet.com domain and will point
it to my updates. So if you already follow me on Twitter (hint:

I've moved recently) or are my friend on Facebook, you'll see the Untappd postings show up there, too.

[Evo's note: That was three years ago. Today I spend most of my time on Google+. So if you feel like following, that's the best place to find me. For now.]

Calling all Magic Fridge supporters...

For those of you who have been following me for a long time, you'll recall something called "The Magic Fridge" from years ago. I'd like to kick that off again, as I have a mostly empty refrigerator just waiting for a chance to shine. Should you wish to contribute to my month-long experiment, contact me and I'll send you shipping information.

Please be advised that there may be laws against shipping beer from your state. I'm pretty sure there's no law against me *receiving* beer, as I've had it shipped before. Wrap bottles in bubble wrap and pack tightly with more wrapping on the box sides (all six of them), and the bottles should make the trip. Please include a note so I can give credit where credit is due. While our grocery bill will go down, our beer bill will certainly go up. Your support—should you choose to give it—will be much appreciated.

Someone get a doctor!

And as I said earlier, I am doing this under doctor's supervision. I'll see Dr. Terry Simpson (MD, FACS) each and every week. Quite possibly at his place while he's cooking up some sausage dish for me. He says he has reindeer sausage. How can I pass *that* up? Terry and I are both skeptics, so we're looking forward to gathering some data on this process. Yes, we realize the sample size is a touch on the small side, but a sample size of one will still gather more data than the Paleo diet has acquired.

And speaking of data; here's where I'm starting:

```
Body Type: Standard
Gender: Male
Age: 43
Height: 5'11"
Weight: 199 lbs
BMI: 28.6
Fat %: 25.3
Fat Mass: 50.51 lbs
```

That's me. Not too shabby. I've never been a thin man or of an athletic build. Hell, not even when I was a kid. But all things considered, I could be in worse shape.

Weekly, I'll post the new numbers. I don't really have a weight-loss goal with this, though Terry thinks I'll shed at least 8 pounds and drop a few percentage points. I suppose that all depends on how well I stick to the plan, right? Here's to hoping.

Wow. All this writing is making me thirsty. Beer, anyone?

2

Doctor's Orders: Why a Beer Diet?

By Dr. Terry Simpson

When my good friend Evo Terra mentioned his desire to go on this special one-month diet, it was initially going to consist of just beer. Beer wouldn't contain enough protein (9.6 grams a day for the six beers), nor would it contain enough other micronutrients. To add some protein to the diet, I suggested he consume a few sausages to fit the October theme, and Evo didn't take much persuading. Plus, it would give me a reason to make my favorite, reindeer sausage, as his inaugural meal.

If you have been influenced by popular press and are aghast at what Evo did, you're probably wondering how a physician could condone such a diet. The answer is simple: *because we needed to know.*

There are a lot of myths about what a person should eat to become fit, lose weight, and generally maintain their health. What we think we know about how the body reacts to the foods we put inside it and what we really know are two different things. Our brains are all-too easily influenced by the latest popular book-based or fad diet, and we assume that the secret is in eating vegetables, or protein, or ... whatever. Such is the fickle nature of conventional wisdom.

If you follow the "protein" diets–such as Paleo or Atkins–you would assume that sausages are okay, but beer should be horrible. If you're a follower of vegetable-based diets, you'd be okay philosophically with the beer, but you could never eat sausages that contain actual *meat*.

Where do we get those ideas, and is there real science behind them? We get them from popular press. We get them from cherry-picking scientific data. And we get them from our own prejudices.

This month, Evo is embarking on a diet that is at odds with the two great themes of American diets; he is not eating "clean" or "pure" foods and is instead eating "processed foods." Therefore, his diet should be doomed to failure.

Here is the problem: Most of what you have read or heard about diets has more baloney than the sausages that Evo will eat. But those diets do make good sound bites. "Veggies are good for you so only eat those," or alternatively, "Cavemen evolved to eat natural food and we have messed up the world by processing food so it has to be bad."

The most dangerous assumptions about diets come from "population studies," where researchers get food diaries from some individuals, look at the overall health of those studied, and then apply those findings to an entire population. Often, it's just bad science.

Here are a few popular ones you may have heard of over the years, along with the myths they've generated.

Seven Countries Study

From the 1960s through the 1970s, cholesterol was offered up as a serious health threat. Both the American Heart Association and the "McGovern Report" (http://en.wikipedia.org/wiki/

George_McGovern) that set national dietary policy in 1977 cited findings from the Seven Countries Study (http://en.wikipedia.org/wiki/Seven_Countries_Study) as evidence for their official statements clearly showing dietary cholesterol is bad for you, me, and everyone else. This study was a subgroup of a larger study that set policy about saturated fat and cholesterol for the United States for years.

Ancel Keys, a physiologist, architected and promoted the Seven Countries Study, establishing the conclusion that serum cholesterol was strongly associated with heart disease. That part is true. High levels of cholesterol in blood show a dramatic correlation with the incidence of heart disease and stroke. Where Keys got into trouble was making the leap that a diet low in cholesterol would reduce heart disease. His first assumption was that dietary cholesterol would impact blood cholesterol, but it does so only very modestly. His second assumption was that saturated fat would impact heart disease, but years of studies have failed to show evidence that saturated fat impacts blood cholesterol or increases heart disease.

But here's the rub: The statistical data from the Seven Countries Study did not back up Keys's conclusion. The Seven Countries study does not explain the "French paradox" (http://en.wikipedia.org/wiki/French_paradox). The French have a diet rich in saturated fats from both meats and dairy, and yet have one of the lowest rates of heart disease in the western world. This paradox could not be ignored, but the study *did* ignore it. Later people tried to invoke the increased red wine consumption as some magic counter to the saturated fat. The other data point the study ignored was the Japanese had significantly increased consumption of meats after WWII and yet still showed a reduction in strokes and heart disease. Today, we know the "epidemic" of heart disease in those decades was more attributed to the increase in cigarette smoking than dietary changes.

Later in his life, Keys recanted his position, saying cholesterol wasn't so important. He then discovered olive oil, and was one of the founders of the Mediterranean Diet. He lived to be 101.

The China Study — VEGETARIAN MANIFESTO

Many vegetarians and vegans cite the China Study (http://en.wikipedia.org/wiki/China%E2%80%93Cornell%E2%80%93Oxford_Project) as *The Study* showing that eating vegetables will reduce not only heart disease, but also cancer. This study was then summarized in a best-selling book filled with conclusions and anecdotes, but no real science. According to the study, residents of rural China who continued to eat their traditional diet showed a remarkably low incidence of heart disease. Working on the hypothesis that diet played a key role, the lead author, T. Colin Campbell, drew blood from people in the villages and then pooled the samples together. (Yes, he took blood from individuals, then mixed all samples together for analysis instead of looking at each individual member of the community with their health issues and their blood chemistries–how a real study should work). Based on the data from a sample size of 100, he came to the conclusion (oddly enough reinforcing his own bias) that those with a diet high in vegetable proteins lived the longest, and that animal proteins were the primary cause of heart disease, cancer, and halitosis (okay, maybe not halitosis.)

The primary flaw of the study is the same flaw in all population studies: *bad data*. In this case, the data of the *actual* causes of death was lacking. Yes, the incidence of heart disease in China is greater than it was 40 years ago. But it isn't because heart disease has increased nor because they are eating more protein. It's because when a person died of heart disease 40 years ago, the cause of death was often recorded as *something else*. To this day heart disease in China is underreported, and in the day when there were no doctors in these villages it was dramatically underreported.

Most of the data in the study, when critically examined, supports the opposite conclusion of the "findings" Campbell suggests in his book. For example, one village had an extremely higher per-capita consumption of meat–twice that of the US population at the time. Yet the villagers had the lowest incidence of cancer and heart disease. These data also showed that the higher the amounts of processed wheat and sugar in the diets of the villagers in the study, the greater incidence of heart disease. Statistical outliers? More like evidence of the null hypothesis.

Here's the reality. People who lived in rural China during the time of data collection were classic omnivores. They ate–and by all accounts still eat–any and all protein sources available. Mammals, birds, insects … If it flies, walks, crawls, swims, or slithers on the ground, it's quite literally fair game. But when asked by well-meaning researchers in stiff lab coats to detail their protein sources? Well … pride is a strong motivator. Self-selected surveys are always suspect. Direct observation paints a vastly different picture.

The Norwegian Study

The decrease in heart disease during World War 2 in Norway is cited (most often by vegetarians) as proof that animal proteins lead to heart disease. Their conclusion? Heart disease went down because Norwegians had less animal protein available to them. But that conclusion is incorrect.

In 1940, Norway was invaded and occupied by Nazi Germany. Over the course of the next four years, the Germans confiscated nearly all the livestock to feed Nazi soldiers. In the Norwegian population, land-based animal protein consumption was suddenly and almost completely absent, while fish-based protein shot up over 200%. Also sugars, flours, and processed goods were highly rationed and hence available only on a very limited basis. During this time the Norske were forced to forage for plants and eat more fish to survive. Records indicate a noticeable drop in death from heart disease during the German occupation.

The popularized vegetarian conclusion is that it was the absence of red meat that caused the rate of heart disease to decrease in this population. However, this conclusion ignores a key fact: In wartime, the chance of dying from other causes such as trauma (guns), pneumonia, and other infectious diseases increases dramatically. People who die from pneumonia miss their chance of dying from heart disease.

But what about the data itself? Does it really support the meat-as-the-bad-guy conclusion? Read this excerpt from an issue of "Proceedings of the Nutrition Society" called "Food Conditions in Norway During the War, 1939-45":

> "During the first year [starting in spring of 1940] the rationing included all imported foods, bread, fats, sugar, coffee, cocoa, syrup, and coffee substitute. In the second year [starting in late 1941] all kinds of meat and pork, eggs, milk and dairy products were rationed"

No reduction in red meat the first year, and not until late in the second year? Then the mortality drop for 1941 cannot be linked to a reduction in animal protein that clearly didn't happen. Hence the obvious question that I ask pro-vegetarians: "So you are telling me that if someone with heart disease *immediately* becomes a vegetarian, they won't have a heart attack?"

In reality, it appears that Norway suffered from increasing fish (a great source of Omega 3 fatty acids). They grew and ate a lot of potatoes, but had a low amount of refined sugars and almost no margarine (I don't know a respectable Norwegian today who cooks with margarine). But that's really not why heart disease went down.

As mentioned previously, heart disease takes time to kill you. *War doesn't*. The increase of mortality from infectious diseases like pneumonia killed more Norwegians during this time than any other time.

Paleo Diet: Cavemen knew better

Until someone invents a time machine, data collection on the daily habits and lifestyles of Paleolithic man isn't feasible. We cannot even make valid assumptions of people who lived during World War II, so imagine the leaps of faith required to conclude what the caveman ate. While there are people left in the world who still gather and hunt as they did in the Paleolithic era, we don't have good data about their overall health or whether they die from heart disease or other causes of death. Keep in mind that most hunter-gatherer societies–of yesterday and today–are ravaged by infectious disease, killing them long before heart disease will. And we certainly cannot conclude that for 250,000 years we were disease free, had few cavities, or lived in the proverbial Garden of Eden, harmonious with nature. This is made up. Totally made up. But it sells a lot of books, and justifies eating bacon.

Strong Heart Studies -– The Pima Indians

When I arrived as a vascular surgeon to Arizona, I was told that the Pima Indians had something special about them, as they didn't suffer from heart disease. This conventional wisdom was so prevalent that a study was created, the Strong Heart Study (http://www.ncbi.nlm.nih.gov/pubmed/2260546), to try to determine what the Pima Indians had that made them immune from today's heart disease. Immunity would not be a bad thing since they unfortunately have the highest incidence of type 2 diabetes in the world. (http://www.ncbi.nlm.nih.gov/pubmed/2260546) As it turns out, closer examination revealed that the hearts of Pima Indians were no different from anyone else's and their rate of death from heart disease was actually higher than that of the general US population.

At the root of this embarrassing conclusion was, once again, poor data collection. This time, on "the most well-studied population in the world." The Pima Indians had been studied for years by the National Institutes of Health, which even had an outpost there for collecting health data. In addition, these Native Americans received their health care from the Indian Health Service, with a hospital on the reservation and tertiary care in the metropolitan Phoenix Indian Medical Center. Even with the backing of the NIH–a fully staffed health service–the statistics collected and recorded were clearly poor. For years they concluded that Pima Indians had a low rate of heart disease, yet their own study showed this was a false assumption from the beginning. So consider this: If the NIH can make such a bungle, then imagine data collection taking place in a third-world country, without constant oversight, without highly trained researchers, and without modern recording devices. You're likely to find hastily scribed pencil markings in record books just a few decades ago.

The statistics about mortality rates from any population survey are suspect. Conclusions drawn from poor data are useless. The common threads in the popular studies about diet are filled with confirmation bias of the authors.

With Evo's diet, we examined not only his weight but also his body fat, total body water, and muscle mass. We also took blood draws to examine his blood count lipids and liver profiles. Based on that data, we were prepared to stop the diet if he took a turn for the worse. (Spoiler alert: He actually got healthier. We'll detail that later.)

Physician disclaimer time: **Do not attempt this diet on your own.** You need a physician's supervision for something like this. We need to examine this diet on many more individuals and get good data before we recommend this without a physician's supervision. Please share this book with your doctor if you're considering something similar. We'll even autograph a copy for you or sign your e-book reader with a sharpie.

3

Day -4: "Beer and sausage for a month? Are you nuts?"

Sept 27, 2011

I spent the better part of today answering lots of questions about my diet. And by "lots of questions," I mean variations on the same theme:

"Are you nuts?"

No, not in a clinical sense. Though I certainly march to the beat of a different drummer. But nuts? I'll leave that label to those who've earned it.

As I've already mentioned, I'm doing this under doctor's supervision. And not in the condescending "as-your-physician-I-cannot-recommend-this-course-of-action" way you might expect. No, my doctor in in full support. Why? His answer comes in the first paragraph of a blog post about our unorthodox dietary experiment:

> *"My good friend Evo Terra is going on a special one month diet–it was going to be just beer but I convinced him to add some sausages (including my favorite, reindeer sausage). If you have been influenced by popular press you are aghast at what Evo is doing, and how can a physician supervise such. The answer is–because we need to know."*

And know we shall. I highly recommend you read the whole piece, especially if you have preconceived notions of what good nutrition is or is not. I know I've been led down the wrong path before. It happens. Science isn't immune to data manipulation or just bad work. But it is rather good at self-correction.

October 1st is just a few days away. I'm looking forward to this! Especially if Terry is cooking …

4

Day -3: A touch of rejection, a lot of support

Sept 28, 2011

Word of my little experiment is getting around. And even though Untappd declined my request[1] to create a badge for drinking along with me during The Beer Diet, plenty of folks are jumping in with support! Like...

- **Brent from PA:** This film director mistakenly thought his state had nothing good to offer me in the way of craft beer. I set him straight and he's busy packing up some goodies to send my way!
- **Charlie the Beer Guy from AZ:** This man literally taught me to drink good beer. Though his work environment isn't quite as liberal as mine when it comes to consuming alcohol during work hours, he's got a system he thinks he can stick to. As such, he'll be joining me in the beer-and-sausage-only diet the entire month!
- **Chris Miller from OH:** Chris recently shed a boat-load of weight. As he's a fan of beer (and a home brewer), people said he couldn't do it. Ha. He showed them. He's modifying the plan slightly to make it more in line with the good stuff he's already doing for

himself. For the month of October, he'll subsist on fruit for breakfast, a salad for lunch, and beer for dinner. Whenever possible, he'll work sausage into the salads. Go, Chris!

- **Thomas "cmdln" Gideon from MD:** Thomas is joining us in spirit, though he's not quite yet worked out what his regimen will be. He is the co-host of the Living Proof podcast, where I'll be a frequent guest next month to document my progress in audio.
- **Chooch Schubert from DC & John Taylor Williams from MD:** I'm still waiting on firm commitments from these gentlemen, but I know they are in somehow. JTW co-hosts Living Proof with Thomas, so he'll be feeling the pressure!

Thanks for the support, guys! And welcome to the sausage fest! No... wait. That didn't come out right. At any rate, I appreciate you joining me for The Beer Diet!

October 1st hits this Saturday. What should I have for my breakfast beer and the kick-off to the Beer Diet?

Notes

1. Hey, I can't blame them. They probably get loads of people emailing them all the time with "make a special badge for me!" requests. But I still love the tool Untappd provides and will use it every time I drink a beer on my Beer Diet.

5

Day -2: The realities of and compatibility with The Day Job

Sept 29, 2011

The reality of the Beer Diet hit a few people at the office a little harder today. A typical exchange went like this:

> *"Really, you're not just drinking beer and eating sausage the whole month, are you?"*
>
> *"No, really. You're **not** just drinking beer and eating sausage the whole month."*
>
> *"No, I'm serious. You **really are not** just drinking beer and eating sausage the whole month."*
>
> ***"No, you're not."***

Er... yes, I am. I fought a little misconception at the day job today. We have an alcohol policy (throw back to the Mad Men-esque years of my current profession) and I'm willing to follow it to the letter. I reminded them that it's not all that unusual for me to have a beer (or two) at lunch, and I manage to get through the afternoon just fine. This will be just like that. Only I'll have a beer in the morning, probably during a meeting. See? Virtually no difference at all.

The team I manage is going to do their own little play-along, documenting my mood and attitude toward them as the month progresses. I think that's an excellent data point to have! But being the cut-ups that they are, I fully expect to have surreptitiously filmed videos appearing in some mockumentary of what it was like to work under The Monster Who Only Drank Beer and Ate Sausage For a Month. That's OK, kids ... bring it!

The Beer Diet is going to be awesome. You can be awesome and contribute some of your local fare—that's quality craft beer or fantastic sausages—if you want to get involved. You can also follow my beer-as-it-happens antics via Untappd. And of course, I'll keep blogging, tweeting, and Facebooking the whole thing as it unfurls.

II

October

"Quaid… Start the reactor." – Kuato

6

Day 1: It begins

October 1, 2011

Well, that was pretty easy. This is going to be a piece of cake![1]

Today was rather busy. I had to fill in for a talk Jeff Moriarty was supposed to give. But he needed a vacation. From not having a job. Whatever. Then my physician decided I needed to come drink his beer and eat reindeer sausage at his house. Fine, I'll do it. And finally, there was the sneaking in of my dinner beer to the theater. My dinner beer I didn't drink because I was watching *Contagion*. Sorta spoiled my appetite. And desire to touch anyone. Or anything. Ever.

But yes, a good day. On to the details:

- **Beer 1: Franziskaner Hefe-Weisse** by **Spaten-Franziskaner-Bräu**
- **Beer 2: Dale's Pale Ale** by **Oskar Blues Brewery,** accompanied by half a mild Italian sausage. Protein, FTW!
- **Beer 3: Porter Czarny Boss / Black BOSS Porter** by **BOSS Browar Witnica S.A.** courtesy of Dr. Terry Simpson & his lovely wife, April. Oh, and their 1-year-old, JJ. Fantastic people.

- **Beer 4**: **Artisan Golden Ale** by **Jolly Pumpkin Artisan Ales,** also courtesy of Dr. & Mrs., with a reindeer sausage. No, not a half. The whole damned thing. Because it was made of awesome. And Rudolph.
- **Beer 5**: **Calico Amber Ale** by **Ballast Point Brewing**

According to MyFitnessPal, that was just under 1600 calories, which is about 100 shy of my goal. Great! I'll bank it for tomorrow when I'm meeting beer judge and home brewer Thomas Vincent and his new bride, Kris, up in Sedona. Rumor has it there are presents. For me!

And don't forget, you can follow along with my beer drinking as-it-happens the entire month on Twitter and Facebook. And yes, you can support my cause by sending me the two things I need this month: sausage and craft beer!

Notes

1. Those are what we call "famous last words". Ask your parents.

7

Day 2: Poor planning

October 2, 2011

Note to self: *Plan better tomorrow.* We were on the road from 10:00
a.m. until moments ago. And I forgot to take food with me, so I
had to improvise. I did OK, though I wound up eating more than
I wanted. All thanks to piss-poor planning. I'll tell you more later.
Right now, I'm tired and going to bed.

Here's a rundown of what I had today:

- **Beer #1: Tangerine Wheat** by **Lost Coast Brewery**
- **Beer #2: Dale's Pale Ale** by **Oskar Blues Brewery,**
  along with some hastily purchased Genoa salami. Hey,
  it's kinda like sausage!
- **Beer #3 and #4: Myrcenary Double IPA** by **Odell
  Brewing Co.** at Pizza Picazzo's, where I found a rather
  tasty sausage-stuffed poblano pepper! Hey, it was
  mostly sausage. Back off.
- **Beer #5: Snake Charmer** by **Oak Creek Brewery** at
  Oak Creek Brewery
- **Beer #6: King Crimson** by **Oak Creek Brewery** at
  Oak Creek Brewery

- **Beer** #7: **Mirror Pond Pale Ale** by **Deschutes Brewery** at The Tavern Grille
- **Beer** #8: **Black Butte Porter** by **Deschutes Brewery** at The Tavern Grille

Like I said: poor planning. But a good time with good friends. More later. When I've slept.

8

Day 3: I lost 6 pounds! Suck it, Paleo Diet!

October 3, 2011

Three days. Six pounds lost.

OK, that's probably not fair. Let me start at the beginning.

One week ago today, I went in to see my physician, Dr. Terry Simpson. My beer-and-sausage-only diet wasn't slated to begin until the following Saturday, but it was a good time to establish a baseline. All that we recorded appears at the bottom of this post.

When I went in today to do a followup, I had lost six pounds, Even better: Two of those pounds were–according to Terry's fancy scale–from fat! That's pretty damned fantastic.

So do I really think that 2.75 days of beer-and-sausage-only caused me to drop the weight? Well... probably not. I'm making the assumption that I was more conscious of everything I ate after seeing Terry a week ago, several days before I went onto the restrictive diet. I've been paying attention to what I eat for a while now, and that's part of the reason for the Beer Diet in the first place.

But to hell with when I lost the pounds. I really don't give a shit. What is important is that *I lost them*. And I'll lose more, dammit!

Terry has a good write up on what's going on on his doctory-blog.

Check it out. I think he said I could kick a caveman's ass. Damn skippy.

Sedona Recap

So as I said yesterday, my planning sucks. But my outcome did not suck, as I got to hang with the fantastic Thomas and Kris, flown in recently from one of the Carolina states. North... South... whatever. I married the two of them a few months back, and they are old friends of ours from when they used to live in Arizona. Amazing how a little podcasting can bring people together.

After we knocked back a few (too many) brews at Oak Creek Brewing and generally caught up with things, Thomas handed me a present: a couple of brews that don't have distribution in Arizona! The Rye Hopper from French Road was the surprise of the two. Very mellow and clean. I'm a huge fan. Hoppyum from Foothill's Brewing was great as well. Matched my palate perfectly. Yeah, Thomas has been drinking with me for a while.

Today's Drinking

I got a chance to try—and by try I mean completely consume—both of those tonight. Ah, friends. Speaking of that, here's the entire day:

- **Breakfast beer: Boulder Bend Dunkelweizen** by **Leavenworth Biers**
- **Lunch beer: Lubrication** by **Clown Shoes** with a half of a jalapeno-cheddar sausage from Von Hanson's. The vast majority of what I eat this month will be from them. Outstanding!

- **Dinner beer**: The full 650 mL of **Hoppyum IPA** by **Foothills Brewing**, again thanks to Thomas! And I also had the other half of the sausage to round out my protein intake for the day.
- **Nightcap beer**: A 22 oz of **Rye Hopper Ale** by **French Broad Brewing Co.**, also courtesy of Thomas. I'm enjoying the last as I type this, so forgive any typos!

That brings my total calorie count to only 1519. And I'm not really hungry. Excellent. This is going well!

Vital Statistics

Here's what the doctor's machine spit out about me today, one week later. Be sure and compare with a week ago:

```
Body Type: Standard
Gender: Male
Age: 43
Height: 5'11"
Weight: 193.01 lbs.
BMI: 27.7
Fat %: 25.0
Fat Mass: 48.51 lbs
```

That's six pounds down, a lower BMI, and two pounds of fat off my ass! Or ... wherever it fell from. Personally, I don't care!

Want to get involved?

Hey, I'm not begging here. But if you want me to enjoy your local fare—craft beer or sausage—then send me some. For you hard-core craft beer fans, join me on Untappd. It's a kick-ass mobile app, and I'm posting each and every beer as I drink it. I'm up to 19 in the three days so far of the Beer Diet! Most of those check-ins wind up on Twitter and Facebook, so feel free to retweet or comment on my status updates.

9

Doctor's Orders -- Evo vs the Caveman

By Dr. Terry Simpson

The fun part of Evo and his diet is not just tracking his progress each week. I also get a vehicle to comment about other diets that are popular in the press.

The first week and he's already down six pounds. That's after one week of a diet where of all his calories come from beer and sausage. My assessment of Evo after this week–yes, he came into my office for an examination–is that he remains healthy, fit, and full of energy. Evo is working hard at keeping his beer-and-sausage calorie consumption to around 1700 calories a day. Since he burns around 2100 a day, he should lose at least a pound a week. Over the course of the month, he should lose about four pounds–but that is making some assumptions that we will discuss.

In one week Evo beat that four-pound predicted loss. Why the big drop? Well, two pounds of the loss come from total body water. I speculated that might be the diuretic effect of the beer. And yes, he indicated he's making quite-often trips to the head. His fat loss is also about two pounds. Those numbers are somewhat exact–which means the weight loss is real.

Will this diet "work?" Yes, much like a thousand other diets based on a similar principle: Limit caloric intake to less than your body normally burns, and you will lose weight.

Let's add a bit of fine print here for the risk-averse among you: More than just putting Evo on a diet, I'm medically supervising him. During this time Evo's cholesterol level, liver chemistries, and a number of other tests will be utilized to make certain he doesn't get into trouble. To add to it, I've asked Evo to take a multivitamin daily and add a fiber supplement. We're also taking a liberal approach to the word "sausage." If Oktoberfest-inspired contaminants–sauerkraut, peppers, mustard, and the bun–encroach on his sausage, he can eat them. What he's avoiding are the side dishes, like potatoes, rice, pasta. And no, sausage pizza doesn't count, either.

In the office today we discussed the major difference between his Beer Diet and the Paleo Diet. In the days of the caveman, most illness was transmitted through water. Beer is highly purified water (thanks to boiling, fermentation, and alcohol) loaded with additional nutrients like niacin, folate, some protein, potassium, B12, and magnesium. And while some will say that any level of alcohol, even the relatively low levels in beer, is evil–it really isn't. I suspect those who say it is evil are those who are the "pure food," "raw," or "vegan" people who possess a self-righteous superiority about people on diets other than their own.

His meat choice (sausage, a processed food) would also draw their ire. While "processed" has a bad name (as bad as an atheist naming their son Christian), think about the meat in a typical caveman diet. Assume your clan is fortunate enough to take down a big bison, wildebeest, or some other huge creature, providing fresh meat for the entire group. Well, it's fresh *that* day. You aren't likely to take down another mastodon tomorrow, so that meat will need to feed your clan for days, weeks, or months. And what do you get without the benefit of refrigeration, salting, curing, or even the invention of flypaper? Food poisoning. Most of the meat will become rancid quickly, causing illness for many and probably killing a few. Still think Paleolithic man healthier than we are today?

But cavemen evolved. Humans became smarter and learned how to process and preserve meats. Sausage-eating man has virtually eliminated a primary cause of early death of the caveman: botulism, parasites, or bacteria such as salmonella. For that reason, Evo's diet will lead to a longer life than if he had chosen to follow a true Paleo diet. Although ... a true caveman-style diet today would lead to more weight-loss in a month than Evo will experience, but only because its adherents would eventually become sick and die from diseases that modern man has eliminated.

Would you trade a processed pork-and-fennel sausage for rancid bison? Would you really give up your bacteria-free beer to drink from a Giardia-infected stream? Me neither.

10

Day 4: Hello, hunger

October 4, 2011

Today's word is: *hungry*. Yeah, today the hunger really set in. It's manageable, but my stomach has declared that the novelty of the prior four days has worn thin.

That's OK. I'm stronger than my stomach. I think.

My brain knows it's getting enough to eat. I'm consuming a fair amount of calories. And it's not like I don't have plenty of reserves lying around my mid-section. It's bringing the body around to what the brain knows that's the challenge. It isn't so bad during the day, mostly because I've doubled my intake of yerba mate. Caffeine makes for a fantastic appetite suppressant. But the evenings blow. I may add in some mate or maybe tea or coffee to take the edge off. But I tend to sleep like crap when I drink caffeine late in the day. There's always a tradeoff.

Yet I remain committed to the Beer Diet. I knew that there would be challenges going in. This is the first of what will probably be a couple of hurdles in front of me. I'll manage. Here's today's intake:

- **Breakfast beer: Great White** by **Lost Coast Brewery**

- **Lunch** was a **Devastator** by **Wasatch Brewery** and 1/2 of a jalapeno-cheddar sausage. Need to change that up tomorrow. Note to self.
- **Dinner beer** was a **Pumpkin Porter** by **Grand Canyon Brewing Company** that I drank at Mellow Mushroom while some inconsiderate people ate pizza in my presence.
- **Snacked** on the other 1/2 of the sausage at home, chased by a **Dale's Pale Ale** by **Oskar Blues Brewery.**
- **The evening** will end with a full bomber of **Perseverance Ale** by **Alaskan Brewing Co.** That, and a cigar. Nicotine helps, too!

Day five is tomorrow, bringing me 1/6th of the way through the month! Someone send me beer or sausage. Follow me on Twitter, Facebook … you know the drill. I'm tired. Hungry. Need a stogie.

11

Day 5: Beer and coffee get me through the day. Oh, and sausage.

October 5, 2011

I did a slight change-up to my intake process today, the 5th day of the Beer Diet, and that seemed to work better. I chugged some coffee at the beginning of the day, and the early addition of caffeine kept the hunger at bay until I could enjoy my breakfast beer at around 9:00. That was made all the more interesting as there was a staff meeting called at that time. At least two of the attendees were a little shocked I was drinking a beer during the meeting.

Lunch came and went without issue. More beer. Half a sausage. The mild Italian sausage is good, but light on flavor. I'll add a little Sriracha sauce to it tomorrow to add some kick. Flavor I need. In a big way.

I worked a little longer than usual, so added another office beer around 4:45 to end the day. The bad news is that I had a consultation after work, keeping me from my final half of the sausage until around 7:15 that evening. That sucked. Hard.

But things got better when I made a a trip to Total Wine for restocking, since I'm running low on my primary food source–beer. Now I have enough to get me through the weekend. I'll need to load up again after that.

Hunger today was manageable, and I credit the large coffee consumed around 2:30. Looking at the numbers, I see I drank one beer fewer than normal. I can't decide if that's a good thing or a bad thing.

Tomorrow a film crew comes to document my diet at work. No, I'm not kidding. Word gets around. I'm sure that will put the office a bit more on edge.

Here are the stats for today:

- **Breakfast beer**: **Dale's Pale Ale** by **Oskar Blues Brewery**
- **Lunch** was a **G'Knight** by **Oskar Blues Brewery** and 1/2 a mild sausage from Von Hanson's.
- **Pre-dinner brew** was **GUBNA Imperial IPA** by **Oskar Blues Brewery,** rounding out my day of Oskar Blues. Love those guys.
- **Dinner** was a consultation with a client, who graciously picked up the tab for my **Isolation Ale** by **Odell Brewing Co.**
- **Nightcap:** I'm ending the day with the other 1/2 of that sausage and an **Inversion IPA** by **Deschutes Brewery.**

I've given up on MyFitnessPal. It's a nice app and all, but I don't trust the calorie numbers for the beers I'm drinking. I could do the math and figure out the calories on my own, but that's a pain in the ass. I'm a simple guy, so I'm sticking with the simplicity of the Untappd checkin. If I average out 6 beers a day and a single sausage, I'm happy to call that good enough. And if any of you want to ferret out the original gravity and final gravity of the beers I'm drinking to give me a true count, have at it. Me? I'm good.

12

Day 6: Angry at the Beer Diet

October 6, 2011

To say my system is fucked up is among the greatest understatements in history. This challenge is significantly harder than I ever thought it would be. Holy shit. I manage to keep it together fairly well during the day, but my evenings are devolving. Big time.

Yet I'm continuing. Why? Well for starters, I'm a stubborn bastard. Ask around. And I also know that this is the proverbial "wall." If I can get past it, things will get better. That's the way challenges work, even when they aren't beer-based. Changing routines is hard; I get that. It just sucks hard how much I'm experiencing that now.

But I shall carry on. I can quit whenever I want, but right now, I really don't want to quit. Even though this sucks. Hard.

Here's what I did today on the Beer Diet:

- **Breakfast** was a nearly undrinkable **Wild Blue** by **Blue Dawg Brewing.** Seriously. What a piece-of-shit beer.
- **Lunch** was a **St. Rogue Red** by **Rogue Brewery** and half a mild Italian sausage. Some dickhead used up all the Sriracha sauce at work, so I had to go with hot wing sauce. Which I don't really care for. Oh, and I had to eat

it during a mandatory lunch meeting. Strike three, and I'm still at the fucking plate.

- It's **0'Beer:30** today. To celebrate, I had a **Desert Amber** by **Sonoran Brewing Company** at Mellow Mushroom…
- which was followed by a **Turbodog** by **Abita Brewing Company,** also at the Shroom.
- **Skeptics & Cigars** started with a **St. Lupulin** by **Odell Brewing Co.** at Robbie Fox's Public House, where I also gorged on bangers, no mash. Don't ask how many. More than a half. Deal.
- I **wrapped** with a **Duvel** by **Duvel Moortgat** at Robbie Fox's Public House.

Now I'm home, outwardly exhibiting much less vitriol than I'm expressing in this post. I hope. You readers, you are my rage release. Enjoy.

Let's try this shit again tomorrow.

13

Day 8: Return of the Beer Dieter

October 8, 2011

Where was I? Oh yes, hitting the wall. Hard. Who would have thought there would be difficulty in a nothing-but-beer-and-sausage diet?

Oh, right ... you people.

But that's OK. My diet. My rules. I am by no means a masochist (sadism is another thing entirely), so a minor tweak to the diet has me back in the game with a vengeance!

Remember that we're doing this for science (and my love of beer and sausage), and that my observations along the way will help in the hypothesis Terry and I put forward. With that ...

Observation #1: All calories are *not* the same.

Not, at least, to my stomach. Or not to the part of my brain that is telling me how my body feels. Months ago, I restricted my diet to around 1500 calories a day, simply by eating much smaller portions. And that wasn't all that difficult, with only a slight hunger that cropped up an hour or so before mealtime. The first week of the Beer Diet, I had about 50 more calories every day. Yet the hunger that chewed through me last week was anything but slight, and what should have been merely a nagging hunger seemed more like hard-core bitchy starvation. That, and I felt like shit. Very much not right. Even with more calories.

So it's not the calories. It could be the increased caffeine. It could the increased beer consumption. But I can feel the effects of those when they hit. They tend to be short-lived. I don't think either of those can be blamed. Here's why:

Thursday night–The Day of Anger–I gave into my cravings and ate more than 1/2 of a sausage. I ate *two* sausages. And I ate the accompanying sauerkraut. I skipped the potatoes offered, rationalizing that side-dishes didn't qualify.

And I slept like a baby that night. I didn't wake up ravenous. For the first time in a week.

So I latched on to the concept and ran with it. Yesterday at lunch, I ate my normal 1/2 sausage. But rather than scarfing it down in 5 minutes and returning to work. I sat there, chatted with some folks, and took another half hour to slowly eat the second half. That's new for me. I'm a speed-eater, as anyone can tell you.

At around 5:00 that evening, I consumed another half a sausage. That filled me up nicely. And then around 7:30 that night, I ate the rest of that 2nd sausage. And as you'll notice below, the beer intake for Friday was relatively low, considering it was #evfn.

And again, I slept like a baby. No waking up in the middle of the night with food cravings. Victory!

Observation #2: You'll get by with a little help from your friends.

On Saturday, I fried up some maple breakfast sausage and settled into an early day-drinking session. The University of Oklahoma Sooners were in the Red River Shootout game against the University of Texas Long Horns. This is one of THE classic rivalries in college football. I'm heavily vested in one side winning. Because #texassucks. I had one beer per quarter and (eventually) four small sausage patties. And OU kicked the snot out of Texas. Why? Because #texassucks.

Glowing in the post-game (and 4-beer) buzz, I crawled onto the Strida and headed over to fellow beer-dieter Charlie's house. He saddled up on his Strida, and we hauled our two over-the-hill bodies the 4.6 miles to The Watering Hole at Whole Foods. Every Saturday, every pour of beer is $4, which is a smoking deal. We both notched up a couple of uniques, began discussing food options, and biked another 3.3 miles to Flanny's. Both of the Johns were happy to see us, and we were pleasantly surprised to learn they were fully aware of our Beer Diet. So much, in fact, that Big John went completely off-menu, preparing for us a sausage appetizer and main course that we thoroughly enjoyed. LJ played "stump the beer drinkers," choosing one of his tap selections for us before we saw the menu. Details on that below.

Biking, beating Texas, great beers, and a reinforcement of how fun the Beer Diet can be. That's what I call a good weekend.

Here are the stats for the last two days:

Friday

- **Breakfast** beer was a **Mocha Porter** by **Rogue Brewery.**
- **Lunch** was a full sausage enjoyed with a **Dead Guy Ale** by **Rogue Brewery.**

- **Dinner** was a quick 1/2 a sausage, and then #evfn began with a **Wet Snout** by **Sleepy Dog Brewing** at Sleepy Dog Saloon & Brewery …
- which was followed quickly by a **Red Rover Irish Ale** by **Sleepy Dog Brewing** at Sleepy Dog Saloon & Brewery …
- and then culminated with a **Dog Pound** by **Sleepy Dog Brewing** at Sleepy Dog Saloon & Brewery.
- About a half hour later, I finished the other 1/2 of the sausage. That's 2 per day.

Saturday

- Since I knew that OU was going to devour some burnt orange, I though it fitting that I consume a **Somer Orange Honey Ale** by **Rogue Brewery** at kickoff for **breakfast**. It's a whole bomber, so count this as two beers.
- The game was in the bag by halftime, so I celebrated with **Estate Homegrown Ale** by **Sierra Nevada Brewing Co.** and fried up some maple sausage. Again, count this beer as two, and an early **lunch**.
- Charlie and I discussed the finer points of the Beer Diet over a **Devil's Ale** by **SanTan Brewery.**
- Then we biked over to see James for a **Saison de Silly** by **Brasserie de Silly** at The Watering Hole @ Whole Foods.

- We tried a taster of the **Orange Marmalade** by **Bison Brewing Co.** at The Watering Hole @ Whole Foods, too. Don't count that. Only a sip. Not very fantastic.
- We wrapped with a **Double Mocha Porter** by **Rogue Brewery** at The Watering Hole @ Whole Foods.
- John's mystery beer was a **Celebrator** by **Privatbrauerei Franz Inselkammer KG / Brauerei Aying** at Flanny's Bar & Grill.
- We tried for a **Camelback IPA** by **Phoenix Ale Brewery** at Flanny's Bar & Grill, but the keg blew. We only had tasters. Which was enough. Nothing special. Don't count this.
- And our specially prepared sausage-feast **dinner** was enjoyed with **Torpedo Extra IPA** by **Sierra Nevada Brewing Co.** at Flanny's Bar & Grill.

And then I went to sleep at 8:00 p.m., crashing out for 12 glorious hours. Looking at the list above, I see why!

The Beer Diet continues. Tomorrow I check back in with the doc. I'll report on my stats as well as give a rundown on my bloodwork. Here's to doctor-supervised craziness!

14

Day 9: I'll see your Vienna Sausage and raise it a Tapatio!

October 9, 2011

I'm marking today's Beer Diet in the WIN column. There were loads of things to do, and all of them were done smashingly well, fueled on nothing but beer and sausage.

The highlight of the day had to be Ruth's *I-passed-the-bar!* celebration, where her mom made me a special sausage dish ... by opening up a can of Vienna sausages just for me! Meant as a gag, they actually paired nicely with an Anchor Steam after they were kicked up a bit by some Tapatio hot sauce, oddly enough.

The next two days will be a bit of challenge. I've got a conference to attend tomorrow and clients to entertain the day after that. Expect massive smuggling to get me through the coming days!

Also, I check in with the Good Doctor tomorrow, so I'll report back on my (or rather his) findings. Here's how today shook out:

- **Breakfast** was an **American Amber Ale** by **Rogue Brewery.**
- **Lunch** was a **G'Knight** by **Oskar Blues Brewery** and the remains of the maple sausage.

- **Dinner** was found at Ruth's party with an **Anchor Steam Beer** by **Anchor Brewing Company** to wash down the Vienna sausage.
- I ended the party with **BridgePort India Pale Ale (IPA)** by **BridgePort Brewing Co.**
- The evening was capped with 1/2 a sausage and a bomber of **Southern Hemisphere Harvest Fresh Hop Ale** by **Sierra Nevada Brewing Co.**

Now to prep for next week!

15

Day 10: Does beer you make fat? Quite the contrary, data shows.

Oct 10, 2011

More great news from the doctor 10 days in on the #BrewDiet, where I subsist on nothing but[1] sausage and beer for the month of October. Survey says ...

```
Body Type: Standard
Gender: Male
Age: 43
Height: 5'10"
Weight: 193.01 lbs
  (exactly the same as last week)
BMI: 27.7
  (exactly the same as last week)
Fat %: 22.9%
  (that's 2.1% down from last week!)
Fat Mass: 44.01 lbs
  (that's down 4.5 pounds! Huge!)
```

If you're paying attention, you'll note that neither my weight nor BMI changed from my initial weigh-in. On the surface, that's discouraging. However, if we look beyond those, you'll see some good stuff. Specifically, I'm converting fat to other sorts of tissue! I'm going with muscle, but hey, it could be a third kidney. I shaved a full two points off my fat percentage, and overall fat mass is down 4.5 pounds. Win!

How much fat can I convert? Hard to say. Well, for me. Terry probably knows. His fancy scale tells me that my fat percentage should be somewhere between 11-22%. I'm just over the high end of that range. Can I get to the middle? Maybe. Hopefully! I think the low end is an unrealistic goal for me. I've never been what you'd call *svelte*, so getting down to 11% would probably require sacrifices and commitments I'm not ready to make.

I still have a couple of more pounds of fat mass to shed before hitting the top end of the desirable range. The scale says I can go all the way down to 18.5 pounds of fat mass, but see my holy-shit-that-sounds-like-hard-work attitude above.

This is going great. Here's a rundown of my consumption for the day:

- **Breakfast** of my go-to-standard and all-time favorite, a **Dale's Pale Ale** by **Oskar Blues Brewery**
- For **lunch**, I tossed back a couple of **Pale Ales** by **Oak Creek Brewing Co.** at Big Earl's BBQ with my good friend C.C. Chapman, in town as an invited speaker at Bolo 2011. Those were paired with a couple of tasty hotlinks!
- **Dinner** was a **Nitro Cutthroat Porter** by **Odell Brewing Co.** and a fantastic brat from Citizen Public House.

- I wrapped the day with an **8th Street Ale** by **Four Peaks Brewing Co.** at Hotel Valley Ho Ballroom as we watched the Vaudeville show at Bolo 2011.

Tomorrow is tricky. I have an off-site client meeting all damned day long. I may have to smuggle a sausage and beer into the bathroom when no one is looking. Make your own jokes.

I'll tell you how it goes tomorrow.

Notes

1. And by "nothing but," you can assume that I'm taking other liquids, like coffee, yerba mate, and water. Nothing with sugar or calories, though. And if the sausage happens to be presented in its natural habitat, like with sauerkraut or on a bed of peppers and onions, it's possible that some (many) of those will be consumed. But I leave off the side dishes. That's cheating.

16

Doctor's Orders -- Who Knew? Beer and Sausage Can Help You Lose Weight!

By Dr. Terry Simpson

This week Evo did not lose any weight. That's it! The diet is invalidated, right? Not so fast. He did, however lose 4.5 pounds of fat. He gained a little water weight (beer is mostly water) and some muscle mass (sausage adds protein, essential for muscle growth) to even things out.

But it's the fat mass we want to lose on any diet. The scale may have stayed the same, but his fat mass, which we measure at each visit with the same equipment I use on all my weight loss patients, has decreased. Fat mass is the stuff that causes the problems. Not just in terms of your appearance or your need for new clothes, but inside your body, too.

Sometimes a doctor should know better: Last week while in Mexico, I had a bad clam. Perhaps inspired by my patient and friend, I enjoyed a refreshing local concoction of fresh clam, shrimp, octopus, lime juice, and beer. It was delicious and I suppose did cause some localized weight loss, as I spent the better part of that day and the next camped out in front of and on the toilet. But had I truly followed the Evo diet (and just had the beer), my chances of getting sick would have been negligible. Beer is highly processed, boiled, filtered, and far more healthy than many drinks you can obtain (including bottled water) from many sources.

The bottom line (I say that a lot because most people want to lose weight from their bottom–I could say "belly line" for some of us) is this: You can and probably will lose some weight on just about any so-called "diet." The trick is losing weight by losing the right kind of mass (fat!) and how sustainable the weight loss is. Extremes are generally bad ideas, and slow and steady wins the race. We know this is an experiment. Evo is doing this under my care–which means I'm keeping him out of trouble. And probably should heed my own advice!

17

Day 11: Of smuggling sausages and beers

October 11, 2011

Well *that* was interesting! As you know, I had the Beer Diet cleared with my employers. My day job is in advertising, and our industry has a history of the three-martini lunch with clients. Not so much in 2011, but no one looks at you funny in advertising if you have a beer at lunch. Or breakfast, I'm proving.

But today was a little different. We had a huge off-site meeting with 50+ individual representatives from our client roster. A catered breakfast and lunch in the ballroom would render me cracking open a beer and whipping out a sausage from my brief-case: rather inappropriate.

Fortunately for me, one of our clients (more than a representative: this guy **is** the client) somehow heard of my diet. He met me at the door with a surreptitiously wrapped turkey sausage smuggled from the breakfast bar! He said he had a beer up in his room. I told him I had a beer in my briefcase. I don't think he believed me. That's OK. I didn't believe him!

Lunch almost worked: a paella, which is traditionally (at least in Arizona) served with chorizo. But in this version, the chorizo was an afterthought, and it would have taken me way too long to pick out just the sausage. And since the chorizo isn't the central part of the dish, I considered that cheating.

So I snuck out–literally–to the parking lot with my lunch bag (hidden in my briefcase) to down a G'Knight and shove half a jalapeno-&-cheddar sausage in my face. I tossed in a few sticks of Trident to keep up the ruse and slipped back in undetected. In my next life, I'm gonna be a double-naught spy!

No one was the wiser. At least I don't think so. If I show up tomorrow with a pink slip on my desk, you'll know differently. Here's how today played out, minus the drama listed above:

- **Breakfast** of a **Dale's Pale Ale** by **Oskar Blues Brewery.** When I got to the off-site, I had a couple of turkey sausages from the buffet. Meh.
- **Lunch** was a hastily consumed half-sausage and the smuggled **G'Knight** by **Oskar Blues Brewery** at Hyatt Regency Scottsdale.
- Came home and enjoyed a **GUBNA Imperial IPA** by **Oskar Blues Brewery.**
- The day wound down with a bomber of **Lips of Faith Kick** by **New Belgium Brewing Company.** Count this as two. And pucker-y.

That's it. Though some out-of-town friends just showed up with a six pack. Work could suck tomorrow. Ciao!

18

Day 12: A monochromatic kind of day

October 12, 2011

I just spent over 12 hours at work, after two days of being "on" at conferences. Any ill effects I might attribute to the Beer Diet are equally explained by anger and animosity.

I'm not good company. With that, here's what I consumed today. I'll shoot for "more chatty" tomorrow:

- Late-ish **breakfast** of a **Japanese Green Tea IPA** by **Stone Brewing Co.**
- **Lunch** was a White Hot from Ted's, and then yet another **Japanese Green Tea IPA** by **Stone Brewing Co.** Rick said he thought I was cheating eating a dog. I told him to eat me.
- **Dinner:** By then I knew I was working super fucking late and asked my lovely wife to bring me a **Japanese Green Tea IPA** by **Stone Brewing Co.** and a sausage.
- **After dinner:** I ate that, then was thirsty again. So I had another **Japanese Green Tea IPA** by **Stone Brewing Co.** Noticing a pattern?

- **After after dinner:** And then I got home and had my 5th **Japanese Green Tea IPA** by **Stone Brewing Co.** of the day.

A monochromatic day, and it's still a damned good beer. Which is the best thing I can say about today.

Good night.

19

Day 13: O'Beer:30 Thursday meets the Beer Diet

October 13, 2011

Today was a good day to drink beer and eat sausage. All hail the Beer Diet!

Though it started out terrible. I've been up since 3:30 a.m. Yeah. That sucks. Especially after yesterday. I couldn't go back to sleep, so I got up and wrote a blog post about Podcamp AZ. Though I won't be talking (specifically) about beer, you should come. It's in November. And I promise you that November in Arizona probably beats the shit out of November where you live..

Let's do the beer and food first:

- **Breakfast** was a **Scotch Ale** by **Boundary Bay Brewery,** with massive thanks to Ryan Gudmundson for supplying me with great Seattle beer! He's provided the theme of today (and probably b'fast and lunch tomorrow!)
- I scarfed down a whole chicken sausage for **lunch,** washing it down with the second helping of Ryan's **Scotch Ale** by **Boundary Bay Brewery.**

- Then it was **O'Beer:30** time with my crew, where I started with a **Kiltlifter Scottish Style Ale** by **Four Peaks Brewing Co.**
- My goal is to eventual march through the all anchor draft options at the beer and pizza place downstairs, so I ended with a **Sunset Amber Ale** by **Grand Canyon Brewing Company.**
- **Dinner** was a sausage-and-salsa stir-fry and an **IPA** by **Boundary Bay Brewery.** Thanks again, Ryan!

And now … I'm fading fast. I stayed up this late doing updates for Podiobooks.com. Man … the chance of me making major screw-ups there are legion this month. So far, they've only been minor. I hope.

So I'm off to bed. As I said, it was a good day. Tomorrow is Friday, and I think I'm taking a half-day to eat up the hours I spent at the office yesterday. And remember: I rarely post on Friday nights. It's #evfn after all, and there's more than my normal amount of drinking involved. I'll see you Saturday morning sometime.

20

Day 14: Boundary Bay Brewing gets it right!

October 14, 2011

Friday is always a good day on the Beer Diet. This one was even better, as I only worked until about noon. Slowly, I'm making up for that terrible long day on Wednesday that we're just going to forget about, OK?

Major props to Boundary Bay Brewery. They hold the distinction of being the first and (as of yet) only brewery to reach out to me on social channels, thanking me for including their beers in my #BrewDiet. These guys are smart and paying attention to the social space. They didn't offer to send me beer or ask for a testimonial from me. They simply chimed in on one of my (drunkenly misspelled) checkins from yesterday:

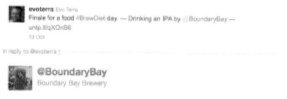

Easy. And smart. Our replies went back and forth a couple of times, and they got exposure to all the folks who follow my antics–many of whom are craft beer drinkers. Their target audience. And you can bet the next time I find myself in Bellingham, I'm stopping to knock a few back at BB!

Here's what I did today:

- **Breakfast** was an **Imperial Oatmeal Stout** by **Boundary Bay Brewery.**
- **Lunch** was a full chicken sausage and the rest of the **Imperial Oatmeal Stout** by **Boundary Bay Brewery,** and so end the fine gifts given to me by Ryan. Of all the Boundary Bays he brought back, I liked this one the most.
- The afternoon found me a bit thirsty/hungry, so I had a pre- #evfn treat of a **Japanese Green Tea IPA** by **Stone Brewing Co.**
- Arrived early at Draw 10 Bar & Grill for #evfn and started off slow with an **Easy Street Wheat** by **Odell Brewing Co.**
- I talked Mel, the cook, into making me a special sausage **dinner.** Again, I'm going way off the menu. It's a good thing JB, the owner, likes me. Washed it down with an **Orange Blossom** by **Papago Brewery** at Draw 10 Bar & Grill.
- Wrapped #evfn and the evening with a **Leg Humper** by **Sleepy Dog Brewing** at Draw 10 Bar & Grill.

Saturday is college football day, which typically increases my beer count. Let's see what happens!

21

Day 15: Mixed-bag Saturday

October 15, 2011

Saturday on the Beer Diet was marked by two disappointing beers, a heartburn-inducing performance by my college football team, and one of the most challenging movies ever.

The bad beers: Shock Top and Oktoberfestier. Read about them below. They have a huge following. I'm in the minority because I do not like them. But I do not like them. Not even a little. But a friend of mine does, so he got a five-pack of the Shock Tops. And the other wasn't even mine to begin with.

The lackluster performance was made by the University of Oklahoma Sooners. It's a good thing I had a birthday party and a movie to go to so I couldn't see the debacle of our terribly-inconsistent-on-the-road team. We pulled it out in the end, but the spread should have been much greater. Gods, I love/hate college football.

And the movie: The Human Centipede 2. Hey, don't judge. I really enjoyed the first movie. And yes, it holds up under multiple viewings. But this? No. Once was enough. Vile isn't strong enough of a word. I'm not upset that I went, as I'm a complete-ist. People were wondering how the director would top the first one. This is how. But it was more of a "bottoming" than a topping. Wow. You probably don't want to see it.

Here is my beer/food rundown for the day:

- For **breakfast**, I thought I'd try drinking a **Shock Top Belgian White** by **Anheuser-Busch,** and what a mistake that was. Yuck. My 2nd worst experience on the Beer Diet. I'm reminded that "popular" does not equal "good."
- Not only did Ryan give me the Boundary Bay beers, he brought back a homebrew. I have no idea what it was, so I just called it an **Unfiltered Wheat** by **Unknown Washington Brewery.** I liked it!
- College football-watching started with a **Session Premium Lager** by **Full Sail Brewing Company.** Oh, and a chicken sausage ...
- Followed by a **Dale's Pale Ale** by **Oskar Blues Brewery.** I was still a little hungry, so I powered through a hot link. Nice!
- I then helped fellow Beer Dieter Charlie finish off his **Oktoberfestbier** by **Spaten-Löwenbräu-Gruppe.** Not what you'd call "good," either.
- Caught the first part of the OU game and a **Session Black Lager** by **Full Sail Brewing Company.**
- Found a solid **HopShock I.P.A.** by **SanTan Brewery** at Ron's 50th birthday party,
- And then smuggled a **Dale's Pale Ale** by **Oskar Blues Brewery** and some Lil' Smokies into the theater

Wow. Well ... it was Saturday, so I'm not all that surprised. And in hindsight (I'm posting this on Sunday), I feel great!

22

Day 16: Of Sundays, sausage, and beer

October 16, 2011

It's day 16 on my Beer Diet. I'm more than halfway through the month. And I'm doing fantastic!

People keep asking me about the deleterious effects of a diet consisting of nothing but sausage and beer for an entire month. In all honesty, there really haven't been any. I do notice pretty severe dry mouth at night. But that's easily defeated by keeping water on the nightstand. Wake up. Drink. Sleep. Easy.

Nor am I sick of eating sausage. Or drinking beer. The variations of both are legion. So if boredom does set in, I just pick up something out of the ordinary. Like when I was at the store today and picked up some sausage that I've been craving. See if you can find it below. Oh, it's going to be a great week coming up!

Today was my lowest beer-intake day ever. That's due to a rather uncharacteristic breakfast. Read on, McDuff:

- No beer for **breakfast**. Instead, I wolfed down an entire chorizo burrito from Filibertos. Because they are made of awesome. Gigantic awesome.
- Finally after noon-time, I started in on the beers. It was bombers for me this weekend, and I started with **Our**

Own Bavarian-Style Doppel Weizen by **Lagunitas Brewing Company.**

- Not to let a good beer die, I finished up with the rest of the **Our Own Bavarian-Style Doppel Weizen** by **Lagunitas Brewing Company.**

- I finally started getting a little hungry and chowed down on a maple-blueberry sausage patty, enjoying it with a **Yeti Imperial Stout** by **Great Divide Brewing Company.** That was pretty sublime.

So that's two (ish) sausage meals and only 4 (ish) beers. Pretty light. Tomorrow is weigh-in day. Here's to hoping!

23

Day 17: Losing never felt so good!

October 17, 2011

Last week, when I saw my doctor for my weekly check-in, I had lost no weight but did drop 4.5 lbs. of fat. By eating sausage and drinking beer, which are the tenets of the Beer Diet. To which my doctor replied:

> *"So to those people who say beer makes you fat: fuck 'em."*

I love my doctor. $20 says you don't get that sort of straight-shooting talk from yours!

This week I'm celebrating continued victory. The vitals:

```
Body Type: Standard
Gender: Male
Age: 43
Height: 5'10"
Weight: 190.51 lbs.
BMI: 27.3
Fat %: 23.5
Fat Mass: 45.01 lbs
```

That's 2.5 pounds down in the week, and a smidge down on my

BMI. But my fat percentage is up by a half of a point, and my fat mass actually increased by a pound. The nascent scientist in me is interested in those increasing fat numbers. And not in a good way. But that sub-personality is way overshadowed by the boy screaming "I've lost nine fucking pounds drinking beer and eating sausage! W00t!"

So I'm going to ignore the fluctuating fat for a while. We're 1/2 the way though this experiment. If Terry has something to say about it, I'll let him. Other wise, I'm going to have another beer. Tomorrow. It's late.

Here's my intake for the day:

- **Breakfast** began with an **Amber Ale** by **Full Sail Brewing Company.**
- **Lunch:** I enjoyed the last of the chicken sausage and quenched my thirst with a **Pale Ale** by **Full Sail Brewing Company.**
- **Dinner** was a hot Italian sausage and a full bomber of **Cali-Belgique IPA** by **Stone Brewing Co.,** so count that as 2 if you're playing at home.
- Wrapping the evening with an **IPA** by **Full Sail Brewing Company.** Which means it's another light night. Ah… adjusting systems.

I'm calling it early tonight. Nice day, I think!

24

Doctor's Orders: S.H.I.T. Beer vs. Craft Beer

By Dr. Terry Simpson

Ask any beer aficionado (no, your slovenly uncle plowing through a case of Hamm's on Sunday is *not* a beer aficionado) and they'll tell you that there is an obvious difference between craft beers and subpar, hoppy-inferior, tasteless (S.H.I.T.) beers. But that difference isn't just in the taste. It's also in the way the body processes different beers. Or so we hypothesize.

As a thought exercise, consider craft beers as whole wheat, and the S.H.I.T. beers as white flour. A person who eats white bread develops a rapid rise in blood sugar, followed by the body responding with high levels of insulin, which in turn converts to fatty acids that end up stored in tissues as fat. (That's how you get fat, by the way. Not from *eating* fat.) Comparatively speaking, less-refined foods like whole wheat cause a lessened and more gradual rise in blood sugar, allowing body to utilize the nutrients and burn them as fuel, rather than storing them for later use (as fat).

Craft beers are less about broken-down, overly-processed ingredients, and more about mixing grains, hops, water, and yeast strains to create an enjoyable experience. S.H.I.T. beers are more about an industrialized chemical refinement that produces a consistent, bland product as cheaply as possible. Our hypothesis is that the body doesn't process the craft beers as quickly as S.H.I.T. beer. And if there's one thing I know about Evo, he doesn't drink S.H.I.T. beer. But you already know that.

Beer has been a source of controversy and misinformation for years. The South Beach Diet (another silly diet plan) claimed that beer was bad for you because of maltose, a much maligned form of sugar with a high glycemic level, meaning it spikes the blood sugar worse than sucrose (table sugar). But any maltose present during the brewing process is long gone by the time the craft beer is ready to pass over your lips–unlike the maltose added to other foods to make them sweeter.

(Doesn't it amaze you that so many diets are based on things people make up? Sadly, it doesn't surprise me, for I know they all are pretty awful.)

Oddly, no one has tested the glycemic index of various styles of beer–craft beer in particular. So Evo and I have a plan to do this. Under physician supervision we will determine the glycemic index of a proper craft beer and a S.H.I.T. beer. After all–this is science, and we are up to the task. I am speaking for Evo here, and he doesn't realize I am going to be getting blood samples from him every fifteen minutes–don't tell him. Just say it's for science, and we'll keep giving him beer.

[Evo's note: Thus far, we've yet to do this. And not because I don't want my finger pricked every 15 minutes. It has more to do with the logistics of getting nine other "volunteers" lined up, some to drink S.H.I.T. beer, some to drink water, and only a few to drink along with me. We're working on it!]

For years beer has gotten the bad rap with just about every diet known to man. It may have started at the turn of the century (the one over 100 years ago, not the more recent one. I wonder when we'll change that phrase? Oh well. A topic for another book at another time) when diabetes was blamed on beer. One also hears about the "beer gut," and all assume it is the quantity of beer that is consumed that causes this physiological condition ... without considering that the other items that are commonly consumed with beer might be the true cause. In this case we know what Evo will be consuming with his beer–not pizza, pretzels or nachos. Just some tasty sausage. Here's to an objective study of a beer diet!

25

Day 18: Death of a Beer Dieter

October 18, 2011

No, it wasn't a literal death. And no, it wasn't me!

But tonight, I was saddened to see this tweet by fellow ex-Beer Diet follower, Charlie the Beer Guy:

@beer_guy
Charlie Toft

Godspeed @evoterra! **Turns out I picked a bad month to radically adjust my dietary intake. I'm officially bailing on the #BrewDiet.**

Charlie hit the wall later in the process than I. He also had arguably a much more difficult challenge. He's in a profession that rhymes with "rule leacher," and they rather frown on daytime drinking. Don't worry: He didn't. But that reduced the number of hours he had available to consume 6-8 beers to get his requisite calories. So it is with a heavy heart that we bid Charlie adieu. I guess I'll just have to bike over to his place and help him get rid of all those extra beers!

Me? I'm doing great! I'm still ecstatic over the results of my doctor's appointment, and I've seen a sneak preview of the documentary video that's being assembled by the fantastic April Simpson. She's made of awesome, so it's made of a similar element! We'll be adding more clips, so I can't show you the final product just yet. But trust me, you're going to love it!

[Evo's edit: Here's that video! (http://goo.gl/1dnfyR)]

I took another blood test today at about the halfway mark of this month. Terry said my pre-diet levels looked average, though my cholesterol is high. I'm not sharing the hard numbers because I want Terry to compare all three sets–before, during and after. If I present them without that comparison, some uneducated asshole would jump in and start arguing why this number is high and that number is low … and I want to avoid that bullshit. We're interested in a change over time, not what any single reference point looks like. That's why I've been doing weekly check-ins on the weight, fat mass, etc. When it's time, we'll talk blood serum levels.

For now? It's time for today's stats, again courtesy of Untappd:

- Trying a little **Coconut Cream Stout** by **Battered Boar Brewing Compan**y for **breakfast**! Way over-carbonated, but very tasty in the AM!
- **Lunch** was a kielbasa and a **Pale Ale** by **Stone Brewing Co.,** possibly the only Stone I'd not yet checked into!
- My late **dinner** was a hot Italian sausage and an **Old Monkeyshine** by **Nimbus Brewing.**
- Tonight's **nightcap** was provided by Mandy, who shared with me one of her favorites: a **Weihenstephaner Hefeweissbier Dunkel** by **Bayerische Staatsbrauerei Weihenstephan.**

That's it. A few loose ends to tie up, and I'm calling it a night. A low-calorie day, really. But I'm plenty full!

26

Day 19: Missing moobs

October 19, 2011

As it turns out, I've lost my moobs. Well... maybe not entirely. But they are significantly reduced in size. I wore a t-shirt today that hasn't been flattering in at least a year. Hey, it may still not be all *that* flattering, but at least there isn't an awning-like overhang between it and my belt.

And speaking of my belt, I moved it up a notch today. That's up, as in tighter. I've got fairly bony hips and no ass to speak of, but something changed, as I was hiking up my drawers all day long. Up one notch tighter on the belt and problem solved. I may go shopping this weekend for 32s!

My son turned 20 today. Happy birthday, NJ. I hope you and your mother enjoyed the sushi I couldn't eat. Not very nice of you. But I love you and expect you to wipe my ass when I'm 90.

Here's what I consumed today:

- **Breakfast** was an **8-Ball Stout** by **Lost Coast Brewery.**
- **Lunch** found me drinking a **Downtown Brown** by **Lost Coast Brewery** and chowing down on a kielbasa!

- Knowing I'd need to brace myself for what was coming next, I had a hot Italian sausage and a **Hoss** by **Great Divide Brewing Company** for an early **dinner.**
- Watched my evil, evil family enjoy sushi while I tolerated a **Tsingtao** by **Tsingtao Brewery** (count as 2).
- Went back to my style of drinking with a **Hop Harvest Ale** by **BridgePort Brewing Co.** (also count as 2).

Tomorrow is O'beer:30 at the office. Who knows what it will bring? All hail the Beer Diet!

27

Day 20: Too much of the Beer Diet?

October 20, 2011

Thursday should be an awesome day of productivity for me after work. My lovely wife, Sheila Dee, teaches classes all day and night at a university, and doesn't return until around 9:00 p.m.. So you'd think that a 9-to-5 wonk like me would get a lot of stuff done.

Except when you factor in O'Beer:30 at my office. My whole team takes off at 3:30 p.m. for an an hour-ish and heads down to the Mellow Mushroom below us to have a couple of pints. Well … that's not true. The Mushroom does 1/2 off drinks on Thursdays from 3-6, so we all splurge and have 20 oz. pours. A couple of times. So it's more like two pints and a half.

And I just discovered that ASH—the Arizona Society of Home-brewers—hits Taste of Tops just a block away from me for happy hour starting at 5:00 p.m. So, being neighborly, I had to stop in. Had to, mind you.

Yeah … I'm kinda done for tonight. Any typos you do not see are purely because of solid editing, I assure you. The first draft was rough. Here's why:

- **Breakfast** was a **Censored** (aka **The Kronic**) by **Lagunitas Brewing Company.**

- **Lunch** was a hot Italian sausage–grilled this time–and a **Maximus** by **Lagunitas Brewing Company.**
- Then #O'Beer:30 started with a **Count Hopula Blood Red IPA** by **SanTan Brewery** at Mellow Mushroom ...
- and flowed into a **Hazelnut Brown Nectar** by **Rogue Ales** at Mellow Mushroom. I did say these were both 20 ounces, right?
- Met the ASH crowd and enjoyed an **Outer Darkness** by **Salt Lake Brewing – Squatters** at Taste of Top's.
- Home, where a kielbasa and too much Sriracha sauce had me pounding a full bomber of a **High Tide IPA** by **Port Brewing Company.** Count this as 2.

So I'm kinda done. Here's to a good night's sleep and a fab day tomorrow!

28

Day 21: You, me, and TV

October 21, 2011

Tonight I was interviewed by the lovely Carey Pena, investigative reporter and fantastic woman on 3TV here in Phoenix. She came to ShEvo Studios with Jeremy the Camera Guy and did a big video shoot that will show up on the news in about 30 minutes. Yay! And just as soon as it's available online, I'll tweet and Facebook it to the world.

[Edit: Here it is! http://goo.gl/aaYR3E]

So here I sit, post-#evfn, post-TV interview and trying to figure out what we're doing tonight. That is completely controlled by the women-folk in my life, so I'm calling it short.

Here's what I drank/ate tonight:

- **Breakfast** found me sipping a **Milk Stout Nitro** by **Left Hand Brewing Company.**
- **Lunch** was kielbasa with BBQ sauce and a **Polestar Pilsner** by **Left Hand Brewing Company.**
- Then Carey Pena came over and made me eat another kielbasa, and on my own I had a **Double Stout** by **Green Flash Brewing Co.**

- Transportation arrived to take us to The Hungry Monk, where I had a **Rotator IPA: Falconer's IPA** by **Widmer Brothers Brewing Company.**
- I kept drinking, heading to a **Kellerweisse** by **Free State Brewing Co.** at The Hungry Monk.
- Not to call it too early, I moved on to a **NorCal IPA** by **Moylan's Brewery.**
- I called it a night—so far—with a **Two Hearted Ale** by **Bell's Brewery, Inc.**
- LATE EDITION! Looks like I wasn't as done as I thought. A buddy of mine with different drinking tastes came over, and we split a **Belgian Style Yeti** by **Great Divide Brewing Company.** Damned tasty!

And now, in theory, I'm off to dance. Tomorrow I'm drinking with the Arizona Society of Homebrewers. That'll be interesting.

29

Day 22: Arizona Society of Homebrewers

October 22, 2011

Today was the Arizona Society of Homebrewers Oktoberfest event. Holy. Cattle.

I finally signed up for ASH, though I'm not a home brewer and have no intentions of becoming one. But ASH is a an organization worth supporting. And as a member, I get to go to their events and drink their beer. SCORE!

Here's how today went:

- Show up.
- Start drinking.
- Keep drinking.
- Eat a sausage.
- Get the wife to pick me up.

Awesome. Dozens of home brews available on a pour-as-much-as-you-want basis. Some were fantastic, and all were very drinkable. Such is the kind of club ASH is: These guys are about as pro-sumer as you get.

I fielded lots of "hey didn't I see you last night on TV?" questions, or affirmed the "Oh, you're the guy drinking beer and eating sausage this month" comments. I was by no means a celebrity at this event that drew in hundreds, but it was nice to be recognized.

I didn't even bother trying to keep up on Untapped. I tried no fewer than 20 beers, meads, and various other libations tonight. Quantities ranged from sips to pints. 2 sausages for the day, and that was it. You'll forgive this post, as I'm a little toasted and need to watch some college football to let it mellow out.

And I've got the sausage from last night's TV spot cooking. Going to be a great week!

_____

Day 23: Sunday, with sausage

October 23, 2011

I ate *way* too much food today.

As I was headed to a late-morning meeting, my belly commanded a stop at Doggie-bertos. You had me at Chorizo Burrito!

Then we went to Citizen Public House in Old Town Scottsdale. They've taken the Sausage of the Day off the menu, but were happy to adapt to my dietary restrictions with a plate full of sausage (and maybe other) goodness!

Also, it pays to know folks. I was introduced to Richie at CPH by local art pusher Dan Semenchuk. That led to a bit of special treatment by the CPH staff, for which I am quite grateful! Significant thanks to our friends Susan & Paul from Los Angeles for spending a great evening with us.

That's my kind of Sunday on the Beer Diet! Here's the intake:

- **Breakfast** was sans beer. Sorry. But damn, that was a fine chorizo burrito!
- **Lunch** was sausage-free (after that breakfast) when I cracked open a 22-oz **25th Anniversary Vanilla Doubledog** by **Abita Brewing Company.** It was very

decent and got much better when I let the second half sit for an hour on the counter before drinking. Don't get this too cold.

- Sundays are bomber days, so I started off with half of a **Danny's Irish Style Red Ale** by **Moylan's Brewery.** A solid red. I like mine more aggressive, but I can deal.
- Waiting for our friends to arrive, I enjoyed a **Ruination IPA** by **Stone Brewing Co.** at Citizen Public House. Bomber. So count as 2.
- **Dinner** was an off-menu extravaganza of sausage, washed down with a **Hefeweizen** by **Four Peaks Brewing Co.** at Citizen Public House.
- Now, writing this post, I'm killing the last of the **Danny's Irish Style Red Ale** by **Moylan's Brewery.**

Tomorrow I visit Terry's office again. I'll have weight results for you soon!

31

Day 24: Sausage + Beer = -2 lbs. of pure fat. Losing again!

October 24, 2011

Monday is check-in day with the doc. It always makes me nervous, and this time was no exception. Largely because of the stupid amount of food I ate yesterday. But still, that was only one day, so only the scales will tell.

Oh, and what a sweet song they sang! The details:

```
Body Type: Standard
Gender: Male
Age: 43
Height: 5'10"
Weight: 188.5 lbs.
BMI: 27.3
Fat %: 22.7%
Fat Mass: 43.01 lbs.
```

If you're keeping score at home, that's 2 pounds of pure fat and almost a full point of fat percentage down from last week. To say I'm a happy camper would be an understatement. I can't remember the last time I was under 190. A decade, at least.

This is going really, really well. Were I a superstitious man, I'd wonder when the other shoe was dropping. But I'm not, and I'm doing all the right things—even when those right things go against conventional wisdom—so I'm happy to keep things going.

I've noticed an interesting banter among people when they learn of my success. I think I'll save that for tomorrow. Here's the intake for those playing along at home:

- **Breakfast** found me in a meeting, drinking a **Messiah Bold** by **Shmaltz Brewing Company (He'Brew).**
- Working **lunch** was an andouille sausage (hot!) and a **He'brew Genesis Ale** by **Shmaltz Brewing Company (He'Brew).** Yeah, the people I work with are officially jealous.
- **Dinner** was a nice Italian sausage from I-don't-remember-where and an **Old Blarney Barleywine** by **Moylan's Brewery.** Count this as 2, since it's a bomber. And a VERY BIG BEER.
- I'll end with a **Ten FIDY** by **Oskar Blues Brewery.** Fitting.

Good night!

32

Day 25: "Your diet would never work for me."

October 25, 2011

"Your diet would never work for me."

I've heard that a few times now. And it puzzles me. Sure, I know I'm a sample size of one. And because of that, I may be a statistical outlier. But if you know anything about stats, you know the odds say something different. Outliers are things you find in a large sample size. I haven't tried this before. I tried it once–and repeated it for 25 days so far–and it's worked. Is there a chance I'm a fluke? Sure. But you'd be a fool to bet that way.

Invariably—and this may get a little on the sensitive side—the people who have said this to me have been overweight. And oddly enough, they've all been women.

And I get it. People who are overweight have probably been through more than one "lose weight fast" scheme before. And they've all—obviously—failed. So here's one more idiot with what ostensibly looks like the novel-est of novelty diets ever. "If that crazy diet lauded over by thousands didn't work for me, there's no way this one can." I get it.

Why only women? It could simply be explained by projected machismo. Boys are supposed to like beer and sausage. Girls are not. No offense, Bavarian Babes, but that's the way it's done over here. So some of the immediate incredulity could have to do with gonads. Who knows?

Regardless, here's what I do know; this isn't rocket surgery. I'm not losing weight because I'm drinking beer and eating sausage. I'm losing weight because I'm putting fewer calories in my gut. The data I'm collecting will ultimately demonstrate that even foods considered "unhealthy" are perfectly fine as long as they are consumed in moderation. I can't say that all calories are or are not created equal. But I what I can say is that it sure as hell doesn't look like calories from beer and sausage are all that bad for you.

But then again, our data collection of this experiment isn't over. Speaking of that...

- A rather late (11:00 a.m.) **breakfast** beer of a **Palo Santo Marron** by **Dogfish Head Craft Brewery**
- For **lunch**, a **Little Sumpin' Sumpin' Ale** by **Lagunitas Brewing Company** to go with my andouille sausage!
- **Dinner** was a sausage medley with a coconut curry sauce and an **Alleycat Amber** by **Lost Coast Brewery.**
- Ended the evening with a **20th Anniversary Imperial IPA** by **Anderson Valley Brewing Company.**

Four beers? Wow. That can't be much more than 1400 calories for the day. And I'm not hungry. Nifty! Thank you, Beer Diet!

33

Day 26: Eye to the future

October 26, 2011

After today, there will be five more entries chronicling my month-long experiment of eating sausage and drinking beer. The end, as they say, is nigh.

At this point, it's a foregone conclusion that I'll finish. Sticking with the restriction hasn't been a real challenge since October 6th. That was a Very Bad Day. But now, my body has completely adapted and continues to shed weight. More importantly, **fat**. Hell, look at my daily intake below! Two sausages and four beers? That's an incredibly low calorie count.

So what's next? Do I keep going, finding the equilibrium point? I can't continue to lose weight on this diet. There exists a point of diminishing returns. If not, I'd be below my birth weight by next Thanksgiving! (Do the math.)

Or do I stick with the low-volume eating (call it caloric restriction if you like), adding in foods I've missed, like pizza? But instead of a whole pie (not all that uncommon previously), have only a slice? But will I be able to keep up the protein level that keeps my doctor grinning? Oh, and my muscle tissue from not being devoured for nourishment.

Maybe I keep the beer intake and mix in the idea of small portions, to see what happens? Do I switch over to scotch? Sake? Maybe mixed drinks of equal impact?

It's a damned fine question. And one I guess I'd better figure out in the next five days, huh?

Here's what I did on my Beer Diet today:

- **Breakfast** was a **Clementine** by **Clown Shoes**. Very tangerine-y.
- For **lunch**, a **Brother David's Triple Abbey Style Ale** by **Anderson Valley Brewing Company** and the remainders of my sausage/curry medley from last night.
- **Dinner** was another Italian sausage from Costco and a **471 Small Batch IPA** by **Breckenridge Brewery**, which you may count as two (I did) as it was a bomber.

Here's to tomorrow!

34

Day 27: Spooky ending in sight

October 27, 2011

It's going to be a busy end to the Beer Diet. Tomorrow is Ignite Phoenix, plus a concert featuring a friend of mine. Zombies, from what I understand, will be the norm. Prior to that, I'm doing my best to draw the ire of Human Resources, wearing what is ostensibly one of the most offensive Halloween costumes. Ever. Seriously.

Saturday we're hosting a combination Halloween party and moving-away party for our old house. The kid is moving out, so it's time to downsize. I'll enjoy the savings, as well as the less cavernous feel. So it's lodging-hunting in the morning, party-time at night. I'll be wearing a different costume that's less offensive. But still a bit odd.

Sunday should prove fairly normal. I've a meeting on e-publishing things, then I'll play catchup on the loss of productivity from Saturday. And quite possibly be nursing a hangover. I wonder how that will be on the Beer Diet? I'll let you know.

And then there is Monday, the final day of the month. It's also the official Halloween, and my team at work are dressing up. Again. With different costumes. Themed. And it's my day to see the doc for the final time, with a final check-in of my stats.

But don't fret. I have a feeling you'll be seeing more of the Beer Diet. I don't think we're quite done.

Regardless, you've got four more posts from me coming. Then probably a fifth telling you what my plans are. This should be interesting.

My intake for Thursday:

- **Breakfast** was a **Monks Wit** by **Abbey Beverage Company LLC**, enjoyed during a finance meeting at work. Because those should always be tempered with beer.
- For **lunch**, a **PILS** by **Lagunitas Brewing Company** and the requisite sausage.
- **Dinner** was sausage plus a bomber of a **Dragoons Dry Irish Stout** by **Moylan's Brewery**, so count as two.
- My **nightcap** (prior to shaving for my Halloween costume, which was probably foolish) was a VERY tasty **Bittersweet Lenny's R.I.P.A. by Shmaltz Brewing Company (He'Brew)**. Gave it 4 stars on Untappd!

Sweet dreams and bitter beer!

35

Day 28: Igniting zombified Zeppelins

October 28, 2011

Fridays are always fun days on the Beer Diet. Typically that's because of #evfn, where more than the normal amount of drinking ensues. This day was fun for a few different reasons.

First, it was our company Halloween party. Half a day at work—in costume—then a beer-and-bratwurst party! Was that a special concession for me? Probably. Very much so.

Second, it was Ignite Phoenix #11. Explaining Ignite to someone who's not seen it is rather difficult. It's an evening where 18 different speakers present their passion, thoughts, and ideas to an audience of some 800. Presentations are five minutes long, and contain exactly 20 slides that auto advance every 15 seconds. To say I'm an unabashed fan of Ignite is somewhat of an understatement. I've presented in this format seven different times and have never missed a show here in Phoenix. Since I wasn't presenting, I could have a beer. And enjoy some sort of sausage feast from Short Leash, one of the food trucks parked outside during intermission. I have no idea what I had, as they use clever names and interesting combinations of sausage types, condiments, and breads. I told the guy to pick for me. It was damned tasty!

After Ignite, we were off to take in a zombified Led Zeppelin cover band. No, not kidding. Hey it's Halloween weekend! Beer at places like this suck by and large, so the pickings are slim. But I made do, and we had a good time with more of our friends.

The breakdown of my intake:

- **Breakfast** was a **Ten FIDY** by **Oskar Blues Brewery.** And no, that doesn't help with productivity. Good thing it was a short day.
- **Lunch** was a sausage, sans beer. Hey, there's a party to go to.
- Party drinks: 3x with an **8th Street Ale** by **Four Peaks Brewing Co.** Not my favorite. But it worked in the setting. Oh, and I might have had a bratwurst. With sauerkraut.
- At Ignite Phoenix 11, I had a **Ponderosa IPA** by **Prescott Brewing Company.** Oh, and that Short Leash meal. Damned fine.
- Nightcapping with a **Pale Ale** by **Sierra Nevada Brewing Co.** at Club Red.

Saturday night is our own Halloween party. I shall do my level best to track the fun!

36

Day 29: Halloween party

October 29, 2011

Today was our Halloween party. Knowing that, I probably should have planned better. In hindsight, I *know* I should have. But I didn't, which isn't all that surprising.

If you've skipped ahead, please understand that this day is rather atypical of the 28 days that have come before on the Beer Diet. But hey, it was a party. So party we must. And did.

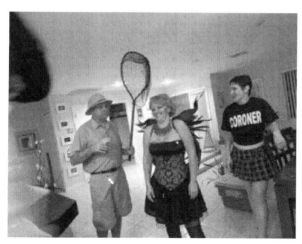

Image courtesy of Debbie Walker.

That's me on the left, dressed as a fairy hunter. Why a fairy hunter? Because my wife dressed like a fairy. And I had to hunt for her. I guess. And say hi to Ruthie on the other side. As a non-drinker, she has mad patience to show up and hang out with us sots. Or maybe we just provide ample entertainment that serves to validate her decision not to drink!

Here's the rundown on my intake:

- **Breakfast** was a **Yellow Wolf** by **Alameda Brewhouse**, plus some nice maple sausage links. It's a bomber, so count two.
- **Lunch** was a **Noël Des Géants** by **Brasserie Des Géants**. Another bomber. 2 more points. Plus I had some hot pork sausage that didn't get used in the dip I made for the party.
- The party began and I started with a **Little Sumpin' Wild Ale** by **Lagunitas Brewing Company**,
- then a **Morimoto Soba Ale** by **Rogue Ales**,
- then a **Brainless On Cherries** by **Epic Brewing Co.**,
- followed by a **Winter Solstice** by **Anderson Valley Brewing Company**,
- … and a whole bunch more I forgot to add. That explains how I'm feeling as I write this on Sunday.

The party was pretty epic. Thanks to everyone who came out. Assuming we're still talking, that is.

37

Day 30: Slow moving Sunday

October 30, 2011

Short day. Short post. Read the prior entry one more time to find out why.

- A chorizo burrito. Fantastic hangover food. When I got up at little after noon.
- Around 3:00, a **Vanilla Porter** by **Breckenridge Brewery**
- Then an **IPA** by **Stone Brewing Co**. at around 6:00 p.m.

And I'm spent. Literally. Here's to tomorrow. The last day (?) of the Beer Diet.

38

Day 31: Last (?) day of The Beer Diet

October 31, 2011

If you've been following me on social media, you already know the score. I'm a very, very happy man.

If you're not following me there, you'll have to wait for the final results. Because in this entry, all I'm going to do is tell you about my intake. They call this "cliffhanging." Deal. The next entry will reveal all.

- **Breakfast** was a bomber of **Irish Red by Rubicon Brewing Company**, courtesy of Katie Charland's husband, Tyler.
- **Lunch** was the rest of that breakfast bomber and a brat I cooked with a not-all-that-great coconut stout. But it made a pretty good beer brat!
- Talked a little biz-nass while enjoying a **Count Hopula Blood Red IPA** by **SanTan Brewery.**
- Post-fantastic doctor visit, I had a hotdog and a **Hop Ottin IPA** by **Anderson Valley Brewing Company** at The Garage Restaurant & Bar.

- Wrapped the evening with a bomber of **Hoppy Feet** by **Clown Shoes**, so mark it down as 2 if you're playing along at home.

And that's it! Or is it?

Oh, and Happy Halloween!

39

Final results of the Beer Diet

November 1, 2011

Well... that was that. Yesterday was the final day of one month of drinking beer and eating sausage. I called it the Beer Diet, and it was a grand time. And it was for SCIENCE!

Thanks to all of you who encouraged me along the way. Extra thanks to those of you who contributed by sending me beer. Much appreciated!

OK, let's get right down to it.

Beer Diet Beer Facts

- **100 "uniques."** That's a beer I've never had before. Or if I did, I hadn't yet put it into Untappd. I started at 308 uniques and ended today at 408. No, that wasn't planned. But I do appreciate the simple math.
- **~154 total beers.** Why the tilde in front? Because let's face it, there were plenty of evenings (like last Saturday) when not all the beers went into Untappd. I don't think I missed any uniques, but I know for a fact I missed plenty of beers. That, and many were bombers which

classify as two. So I'm betting the number was closer to 200. 200/31 = 6.5 beers a day. Sounds about right.

Beer Diet Sausage Facts

- ~62 sausages. Again with the tilde. Look... most days I had two. On rare occasion I had more than that. But for the first 6 days, I only had one. Were we really in a super-detailed, double-blind study, I'd have it a tad more exact. But we're not, so I'm doing the easy math of 2 x 31 for the answer.

OK, that's the intake. What about the results? I think you'll be pleasantly surprised. I know I was.

Weight Loss Facts

First, let's set the baseline. This is important to those of you keeping score at home. None of these things changed in the last 31 days:

```
Body Type: Standard
Gender: Male
Age: 43
Height: 5'10"
```

But here's what did change. I'll give you before and after numbers from the doc's fancy scale:

```
Original Weight: 199.0 lbs
Ending Weight: 185.1 lbs
```

Here, let me help you with that math: that's a loss of 13.5 pounds! Fuck it! I'm rounding up! 14 pounds LOST. Eating sausage and drinking beer!

But hey, that's just weight. We all know that weight changes with fluid. Is it all that surprising? Let's look at the rest of the numbers:

```
Original BMI: 28.6
Final BMI: 26.6
```

That's a net loss of two for my BMI. I'd be more excited, but I don't know what BMI means. But it's down by two, so that sounds good to me. If you care, look it up. If you know, good for you! I don't care. Don't bother telling me. Because I don't care. *[Editor's note: Rats. I was all ready to tell you. But now I won't. So there. Nyah.]*

```
Original Fat %: 25.3
Final Fat %: 21.4
```

OK, I'm smart enough to figure out percentages. That means that I dropped a full four percentage points (rounding up, remember?) of my mass as pure, nasty fat. That sounds pretty fantastic. And according to the "target" numbers on my doctor's fancy scale, that's within the "desirable range."

Didja hear that? I'm *desirable*!

But let's not get ahead of ourselves. That fat % number translates directly to fat mass:

```
Original Fat Mass: 50.5 lbs
Final Fat Mass: 39.5 lbs
```

If the term "fat mass" doesn't sound nasty to you, what the hell is wrong with you? *I've dropped 11 pounds of fat mass!* And if I were to travel to the moon, those 11 pounds of mass would still be gone! I love physics![1]

But you're not a physicist. You know what the scales tell you. And those scales would say something different on the moon. And I'm not likely to travel to the moon. Ever. Which kind of sucks. But I'll get over it. Why? Because I lost 14 pounds eating sausage and drinking beer!

Yeah, yeah … some of you want to know about my cholesterol, lipids, and other funky blood serum stuff. I'm going to let my doctor discuss those results. Suffice to say that I'm not dropping dead anytime soon. In fact, my panel looks better than when I started. No, I'm not kidding. Stay tuned for that.

What's next? Well, I'd like to keep it off, obviously. But I'm also ready for other things to eat. Maybe I'll do this on a regular basis. I have some ideas … and this isn't over!

Notes

1. Sadly, this isn't true. Well, the part about me loving physics is. But the fancy scale in Terry's office uses mass in a more colloquial term. It's still weight and therefore totally reliant on local gravity.

40

Doctor's Orders: Beer Diet Results

By Dr. Terry Simpson

Who would have imagined that my patient Evo would have lost 14 pounds on the "beer and sausage" diet (which I'm now calling the Evo Diet and recommending to my patients) in just a month?

(Just kidding. I'm not recommending this diet to my patients or anyone else. This was a fun and interesting experiment between two friends, where I was happy to provide intensive oversight and supervision. As our friends the Mythbusters will tell you: Don't try this at home.)

Based on the evidence collected, the effects of the Evo Diet are seen in more places than just on the surface. Comparing his blood serum levels throughout the program (we tested before, during, and after), we noticed some significant changes. Let's put these in bullet-point form so they are easy for you to remember.

After 31 days of sausage and beer as his sole calorie source:

- His triglyceride level dropped by half.
- His cholesterol dropped by a third.
- His "good" cholesterol increased.
- His liver enzymes showed no significant changes.

Keep in mind that the 14 pounds he lost was more than just "weight." His fat mass dropped most of all, and the only non-fat mass of his that decreased was that tissue associated with and supporting the fat mass. (Yes ... I know. That sounds complicated. It will make sense to your doctor.) His muscle mass maintained itself, which I attribute to the protein ingested from the sausage. A wise addition from his original plan to consume only beer, which would have placed him in a severe protein deficit.

There is one important thing to keep in mind: We do not know enough about science and medicine and diets to be able to say anything to anyone about which diet is healthy and which is not. Yes, that's true even with this example, where we collected more data points for this single month of the Evo Diet than Ornish or any other "weight loss guru" ever bothered to do for their diet program.

The Ornish diet is an ultra-low fat diet, under the assumption that fat causes heart disease. The diet is another call to arms for vegans and vegetarians who try to convince omnivores that the Way of the Plant leads to a better life. The famous Ornish line is that his data showed a decrease in "plaques" of patients who had heart disease. When plaque builds up in coronary arteries, the rate of blood flow to the heart is decreased. If one of those plaques becomes unstable, a plug can form in that artery ... and you have yourself a heart attack.

What Ornish did was measure the size of the narrowing of the coronary artery (the plaque size). He noted that after a period of time on his diet these plaques decreased in size by about three percent. That's a pretty small number in a pretty small vessel. If you put a coronary x-ray in front of ten cardiologists and ask them to give you actual size of the artery, their predictions will vary by more ten percent. Yet Ornish and his group managed to have better accuracy with inferior technology over 20 years ago? Color me skeptical.

The Ornish study was based on fewer than 20 patients, including the control group–not what is typically understood to be a statistically relevant sample size. He has since repeated poor data collection with his "research" into prostate cancer and aging, as well.

The data Ornish collected isn't as comprehensive as the data we generated in one month from the Evo Diet. Nor does the Ornish group have as good a result after one month as Evo did. One could assume that we would find people would do better not following the Ornish Diet, but instead following the Evo Diet. This is said with a smile, because the popular press continues to advocate the Ornish diet, which relies on poor data from 20 years ago and has yet to be reproduced. Or on the China Project and its misuse of poor data, that is still cited as evidence that one should become a vegetarian. Evo was not a vegetarian. He didn't follow Ornish. Yet in one month he did better than any have done on those diets in the same time span.

The second important part of Evo's diet was this: There was a simple and yet profound control of his portion sizes. His intake was measured, tracked, and regulated to around 1700 calories per day. It was probably because he was (mostly) able to keep that significant caloric restriction going day after day that Evo lost more than we would expect. Why do I say "probably?" Because even though I am a doctor, with many years of experience with literally thousands of weight-loss patients, I honestly have no clue why he lost so much weight. I knew that he would lose weight, but I could not predict he would lose this much. See my earlier comment about what we simply don't yet know.

What you can take away from Evo's experience is this: First, any successful diet should start by strictly regulating portions. Portion control is a key for any weight loss, including weight loss surgery. Limit your portions, and thus your calories, and you should lose weight. The advantage of beer and sausages is that they come in discrete–and tasty–units that you can easily portion and measure.

What you should not take away from is this that we are recommending beer and sausage as "diet foods." Beer and sausage are not "diet foods." Beer and sausage were, in this case, tools to control portion size. And remember, Evo ate more than just sausage. He ate what came with it. When I cooked for him, he had the peppers and onions that went with my famous reindeer sausage recipe–you can find that recipe and many more on terrysimpson.com. He had bread (yes, I know some of you think bread is the devil's tool) if it came with the sausage. But mostly, it was beer and sausage, in modest portions. Comparatively speaking, that is. Most people wouldn't consider four to five beers a day "modest." But in his case, with a willing place of employment and an extremely patient and designated-driving wife, it worked.

The most important message: We don't understand food as well as Ornish, Atkins, or any other diet guru would have you believe. Be skeptical of anyone who tells you otherwise. And send them a copy of this book as evidence!

III

The Future

"You met me at a very strange time in my life." – Tyler Durden

41

The Beer Diet, Three Years Later

First of all, I hope you've enjoyed the book. I certainly had a great time revisiting (and cleaning up) those old blog posts, reliving the moment.

Throughout the book, I alluded to the chance I might go on with the diet. Well ... I have. Sort of. On this and three other occasions, I've made beer the primary source of calories for me for one month. I repeated the beer and sausage diet in October 2012 and lost 18 pounds. Then I switched sausage for eggs in April 2013. That netted me 14 pounds. And I still haven't had a hard-boiled egg since. [shudder] And as I type this, I'm nearing the halfway point in October 2013, once again on the sausage-fest. No ... wait. That came out wrong. But you know what I meant.

Every time I've done it, I come out with the same—or at least very similar—results: I'm healthier after than when I started. It's not a fluke. It's not a trick. And yes, you can do it. Or something very similar.

Look, I'm not doing this to be some sort of role model. Hell, I'm not any kind of model. I'm just a guy who had a crazy idea, found the right support system, formulated a plan, and then followed it. Pure and simple.

Should you do this? Only if you want to. Or maybe if you're curious. And a little nuts.

Everything I wrote in this book is 100% true, or at least as close to truth as my mind will let me. I wrote it down either the day of or day after the events took place, so there's nothing lost to antiquity. There may be some hazy moments, but I at least took the time to record food as it went in my body. Any reports as to the entertainment of those around me? Highly suspect.

Thanks once again for reading the book. If you struggle with your weight, I highly recommend getting in touch with my doctor and very good friend, Dr. Terry Simpson. And if you'd like to toss back a beer, get in touch with me. If you want to toss back a beer and enjoy a fine cigar at the same time, meet us at the Doc's house some Saturday evening.

Cheers!

- Evo

About Evo Terra

Evo Terra: Publishing. Science. Craft Beer. Not necessarily in that order.

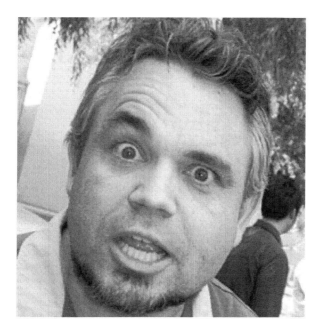

Evo Terra is ... eclectic. Over the years, he's been a nationally syndicated radio show host, professional public speaker, digital business strategist, skapunk bassist, author, hockey coach, mentor, haunted house denizen, farmer and skeptic. He digs *starting* things and is the co-founder of Podiobooks.com, founder of #evfn, co-founder of ePublish Unum, and the originator of The Beer Diet!

When he's not drinking, he writes books. He's the co-author of Podcasting for Dummies and Expert Podcasting Practices for Dummies (yeah, stupid title), the author of Making Killer Google+ Profiles; A Modern Indie Author's Guide, and the author of Writing Awesome Book Blurbs; A Modern Indie Author's Guide. For now.

All that aside, he's made most of his living as a digital business strategist for over a decade. In short, he helps his clients figure out what not to do. He's well versed in what doesn't work, having survived the ups and downs of advertising, retail, publishing, radio, social media and startups.

And he's a lot less of a windbag than his doctor, as you're about to find out.

About Terry Simpson

Terry Simpson, MD: Cook, Scientist, Author, Surgeon

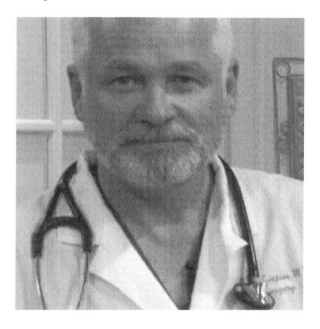

Dr. Terry Simpson resides in Phoenix and his great passions are cooking, research, writing, surgery, and above all, his son. He received his bachelors, masters, and medical degree from The University of Chicago . He has authored a number of scientific papers, as well as books, and a few blogs. His current area of research involve the hypothesis that teaching patients to cook becomes the ultimate lifestyle change for people – and a bit about diets.

Dr. Simpson, when not doing research – can be found in the operating room where he sees a small, but select group of patients. While he performs weight loss surgery, his first rule for his patients is that they make changes to their lifestyles. "I spend more time teaching them to cook than I do operating on them. " He has developed Weight Loss Fest, where his theme is for patients to adopt a better lifestyle by cooking better and more interesting foods. Dr. Simpson also examines diet plans from others with a skeptical, educated eye.

Dr. Simpson is deeply involved in Alaska Native affairs, currently sitting on the board of the Alaska Native Regional Medical Center, and South Central Foundation, a primary care center, where he advocates for better health care for all Alaska Natives. The primary care center they run has won many awards, most recently the Baldridge Award, and is often cited as an example of how primary care centers should be run (during normal hours patients can see a primary care physician within 30 minutes).

Born and raised in Ketchikan, Alaska, the salmon capital of the world (he once hated salmon – -but now loves it, fresh and wild like he enjoys most things), his family goes back 10,000 years, coming to Alaska over the ice bridge on their way to Arizona for the winter. That makes him an Alaska Native (Athabascan variety). His grandfather came to Alaska in the 1890's and his dad was mostly raised in an orphanage in Seward (wrote a book about those experiences – **Jesse Lee Home: My Home** by James L Simpson). His dad and mom have been married for over 60 years, and retired to Oregon. Terry's brother still lives in Alaska – Copper Rail Depot in Copper Center, Alaska (where, like the rest, has authored a book). His mom is a "wizard" in the kitchen – and passed on her love of cooking.

Dr Simpson's true loves are his wife, April, his son, JJ (born 7-20-2010), and his dog, Lucky.

Food Philosophy

I like fresh. When I hear people talk about "local" I think thank goodness for FedEx and UPS – who have made the idea of local about 5000 miles. Growing up in Alaska local was game, fish, and berries but not a lot else. When you write about food, and become skeptical about diets, or lifestyles, you find all sorts of people questioning the basis of your belief.

If you wear a tin hat (meaning you think I want you to have surgery instead of eat well) read this:

Those with tin-hats will say that since I make a part of my living from doing weight loss surgery that I would oppose a diet that would make people thin. Almost like I am a part of "Big Pharma." Let me say this: I don't work for big pharma, or the meat industry, or the dairy industry – I work for the scientific-method. I believe a patient must have a lifestyle change, not just have surgery. Without lifestyle changes weight loss surgery is useless. I spend more time teaching my patients how to cook and make food than I do performing surgery on them.

If you are an animal rights activist then read this:

I do not condone abuse of any animal, in any form. But I do eat meat. I have no issue with an animal giving its life so I can enjoy eating it. I prefer grass fed beef to corn fed beef. Wild salmon much more than farm-raised salmon. You want to send me scary pictures of animals being abused, or films – know that I oppose animal abuse – but animals, as well as plants, have to die in order for me to eat.

If you think you should only eat meat, or only eat vegetables read this:

Humans are flexitarian, not strict carnivore and not vegans. You may follow some guru who only eats meat, or only eats plants- and they may have some anecdotal data about how well they and their followers are doing – but I am not their apostle, and when it comes to research in nutrition, eating, I follow simple and strict evidence based medicine.

But I respect you

I respect those who follow a whole plant diet, as well as my paleo friends. We all have our quirks- but hopefully my view is something you can respect also. I am more than happy to have a debate about any issue in the comment section of my website.

More about his research:

One of Dr. Simpson's favorite pieces from his early work in molecular engineering was:

Post, L.E., Norrild, B., Simpson, T., and Roizman, B. (1982). Chicken Ovalbumin Gene Fused to a Herpes Simplex Virus Alpha Promoter and Linked to a Thymidine Kinase Gene is Regulated Like a Viral Gene.
Molecular and Cell Biology, v.2(3), 233-240.
http://www.ncbi.nlm.nih.gov/pmc/articles/PMC369781/

This represented the first time a non-prokaryotic gene was changed and regulated by a viral gene. Dr. Simpson spent many fun years in Dr. Roizman's laboratory, but discovered he loved people as much as research. Because of being involved in genetic engineering, he has a unique view of genetically modified foods.

He spent a number of years doing vascular surgery- where developing a love for keeping arteries free of disease and found patients who developedan interest in lifestyle changes did much better. This work was inspired when he was a surgeon for the Indian Health Service, and performed vascular surgery among the Pima Indians. While many said these Native Americans didnt have heart disease or vascular disease, Dr. Simpson showed they indeed had it in abundance:

Simpson, T. (1993). Peripheral Vascular Disease Among Native Americans: Pitfalls of the Vascular Examination in Patients with Diabetes.
The Provider, March.
http://www.ihs.gov/provider/index.cfm?module=az_index_1993

He still had some fun with trauma surgery – as in this paper where he wanted the name to be changed to something else, but the editors wouldn't let him.

Phillips BJ; Matthews MR; Caruso DM; Kassir AA; Gregory MW; Simpson T (1998). Tension colothorax: a pleural effusion?
J Trauma, June, 44(6), 1091-1093.
http://www.ncbi.nlm.nih.gov/pubmed/9637169

As vascular surgery and laparoscopic surgery changed Dr. Simpson decided to focus on weight loss surgery, diet interventions, and hoping to help patients avoid vascular issues. He has been the medical editor for Obesity Magazine and now is working on several research projects:

- Low BMI study- for patients who have a lower BMI but request weight loss surgery
- Plication study – a new form of weight loss

- Dietary interventions and weight loss- examining various modular diet plans

He is also working on some bench research, checking levels of appetite hormones in rats, and hopefully people. The hormonal changes of weight loss, and how the weight loss procedures, and diets, alter the changes in hunger hormones.

Mostly he is always looking for new recipes, and trying to pass the love of cooking on to his son.

Made in the USA
Charleston, SC
17 November 2013